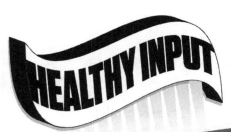

AMERICA'S LEADING DENTISTS

REVEAL THE

SECRET TRUTHS

TO A

HEALTHY BODY

STARTING WITH WHAT YOU

PUT IN YOUR MOUTH

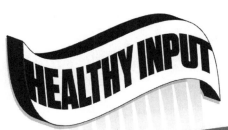

AMERICA'S LEADING DENTISTS

REVEAL THE

SECRET TRUTHS

TO A

HEALTHY BODY

STARTING WITH WHAT YOU

PUT IN YOUR MOUTH

CONTENTS

CHAPTER 10
HEALTHY GUMS, HEALTHY BODY:
THE POWER OF LASER TREATMENTS

CHAPTER 1

DO YOU TRUST YOUR DENTIST?

BY CHRIS GRIFFIN, DDS

I suppose it's easy to question your doctor these days. The ready availability of medical information and disinformation on the internet and in various other places has given people, who normally would always heed their dentist's advice, reason to pause and question. Recently, the profession I love has come under a few attacks from people who question the motives of individual dentists around the country. Some have charged dentists with putting monetary policy above the best interest of their patients.

Please let me pull back the curtain a little bit from the perspective of your local dentist and give you true insight from the other side of the chair. The path your dentist took to be your dental health care provider started way back, a long time ago. It started when they were still a teenager. Your dentist may or may not have been at the top of their class in high school, but once they set foot on college soil, that changed.

As dental schools these days have many multiples of applicants who would love a spot in one of their limited incoming classes, they must divide out the best candidates from the lesser candidates in some fashion. Since they don't personally know each applicant and they can't look into the future, one of the only ways they have to predict which candidates they choose is to look at their grades in college.

Some classes are worth more than others, organic chemistry comes to mind, but a person's entire college transcript is considered. That means that your dentist never was the student who just "got by." It is highly unlikely that your dentist ever slept in after a long night out having fun with their friends at the local bar or hangout in their college town.

Your dentist was home studying most nights possible so they would get that A in a class where it was very unusual to get an A. Your dentist didn't have time to "find themselves." They were focused and pursued the very best in academics for all their years in undergraduate studies.

What about extracurricular activities? Since there are so many students who apply to dental school who did get those near-perfect grades, there is a good chance that your dentist also did more in college than just ace their tests. There is a good chance that they went out into the community to do goodwill type service. They may have gone to help tutor underprivileged kids. They may have helped in local science classes. They may have volunteered at clinics. Many of them spent tens or hundreds of hours working in dental offices for free just so they could say they had some experience. There wasn't time to goof off.

Let's assume that they somehow made it through the minefield of the application process and were accepted into school. When they went to orientation, they were hit with the reality that they would be expected to carry the heaviest load of intense courses imaginable during their first two years. They would easily put in as many hours in class, workshop, and study time as two full time jobs. They would also be expected to master many types of medicine that they would never practically use.

They would be expected to learn all about the nerves of the body. They would be expected to pass Gross Anatomy with flying colors – no matter how squeamish they might be about studying a real human being up close and personal.

Along the way your dentist was asked to pay thousands and thousands of dollars for these rights of knowledge. They spent that money and they spent all their free time away from their friends and loved ones. Even if they were married, they spent way too much time away from their spouse. It is a wonder that any married dental students stayed that way with all the mental and physical demands during those years.

In the later years of dental school your dentist was also expected to start treating real patients in clinical settings with the skill of a seasoned veteran, even though they had very little experience. They managed to fight through all that pressure and found a way to perform up to the lofty standards their professors expected with poise. They found a way to convince their professors to give them their blessing to go out into the real world even as those same professors told many of their peers that dentistry just wasn't for them. Your dentist became such a skilled practitioner that they were allowed the honor of receiving a degree and a license to treat you and others in your community.

When it was all said and done, your dentist spent at least eight years of their life after high school doing the things that other people weren't willing to do, and making the sacrifices that others weren't willing to make – so they could become your dentist.

With all those classes in dental school that taught your dentist everything from human physiology to neurology, the one thing they never taught your dentist to any major degree was just how to make a living performing dental procedures. It is a shame that so many dental schools nitpick their graduates over the most minute and seemingly unimportant clinical details, but leave them to figure out how to run a successful small business on their own.

If your dentist were average, they probably owed much more than a hundred thousand dollars the day they graduated from dental school. If they now own their practice, that means that at some point and time, they took another leap of faith and borrowed some more money to allow themselves to build a place where they could do dentistry and treat patients like you. As you can imagine, dental supplies and equipment are very expensive to purchase and maintain. Still, your dentist loves this profession and they are proud to offer their patients the very best, no matter the cost.

You may see a beautiful office and a nice, professional staff. What you don't see are the risks that your dentist took along the way to be able to provide you with a great experience. Your dentist took a risk when they were young and working hard instead of recreating. They took that risk with absolutely no assurance that they would ever make it to the next step.

Your dentist took a risk by taking on a heavy debt and sacrificing personal time and time with their family and friends with absolutely no assurance that they would actually graduate with a dental degree. Your dentist took a risk by opening a practice with more debt and absolutely no assurance that a single patient would ever walk through their doors. If that had happened, who knows how those huge bills would ever have gotten paid.

To top it off your dentist is obligated to uphold the loftiest of ethical and professional standards. To hold a license in any state, your dentist is held to a code of conduct and honor. They must always treat their patients to the utmost professional standards or they wouldn't be allowed to practice in your town.

Then, your dentist goes above and beyond that standard to make your life better.

Did you know that dentists are the ones who have fought and continue to fight every day to help establish all kinds of programs that prevent cavities? Tell me this. Just how many professions do you know that spend their hard earned money and time trying to prevent the thing that makes them the most money? Cavities lead to all manner of ways that dentists can make money. Whether a dentist does a filling, a crown, a root canal, or an extraction, all those conditions started with a simple cavity. You would think that dentists would be out there passing out sugar and candy to every 3 year-old in America. Instead, your dentist and others are always waging a war against practices that lead to children or adults getting those cavities in the first place. If dentists had their way, all cavities would be eradicated and dentistry, as we all know it, would cease to exist.

Now, consider the pressure that dentists are under when they do treat their patients. People expect perfect results now more than ever, and many times they are looking for someone to blame when those results don't measure up to their expectations. We all know that perfect results are often impossible and many times subjective. Still, every day dentists are out there trying their dead-level best to get their patients the most perfect results possible. Today's dentist is under pressure to perform and succeed in ways your father's dentist never had to face. All this can lead to levels of stress that are easier for some to manage than others.

Hopefully, I have opened your eyes a little bit about the kind of person your dentist really is. That is also the reason I am disturbed when I read some in the media periodically trying to portray average dentists as greedy people looking out for their own interests at the expense of their patients. While I am sure that out of the over one hundred thousand dentists practicing in the United States, there are bound to be a few bad apples, chances are that your dentist is truly one of the good guys.

Your dentist takes pains to find the best treatments for you by taking hours and hours of continuing medical education each year. Your dentist spends money that could have gone into their bank accounts to invest in the best new equipment that they know will make your dental experience better. Your dentist always tries to consider all the possible options for your needed treatment, even if you try to persuade them to do what you want.

Your dentist knows that they have to make those hard decisions and risk making you, the patient, unhappy with them when they advise against your requests. Your dentist always strives for that elusive perfection, even though they know it is unattainable and you don't. Your dentist still tries. Your dentist rarely goes through an entire weekend without working in some way, shape, or fashion. Whether it is coming in to the office to see a patient with an emergency after hours or phoning in a prescription to a pharmacy for one of their patients. Your dentist never truly gets away from being a doctor.

How many of those who criticize and cast a bad light on this profession would want to give up their free time in such a way? How many of these people would give up their anonymity to continue to serve? Just keep all of this in mind the next time you hear someone making a disparaging remark about your dentist.

The truth is that your dentist is quite an exceptional person and your community is a better place with them a part of it. They are certainly worthy of your trust.

Just think of all the things that you know your dentist does to help people. Then multiply that several times to get an idea of all they really do because you would never know about many of the charitable causes your dentist supports or participates in. Your dentist has given back so much and accomplished so much in their careers that they could easily fill the pages of a book.

Just don't expect your dentist to brag on themselves about all their accomplishments. That's just not their way.

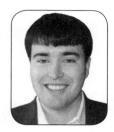

About Dr. Chris Griffin

Chris Griffin, DDS graduated from the University of Tennessee in 1998 with a DDS degree and began solo practice in Mississippi in 1999. By 2003, he received a Fellowship in the Academy of General Dentistry at the age of 29, and became the youngest person from Mississippi ever to receive the FAGD award at that time. During this pursuit, Dr. Griffin acquired many different general dental skills, like sedation and orthodontics, and brought them to his hometown community of Ripley, MS.

In 2008, Dr. Griffin founded the Capacity Academy to help other dentists learn the most efficient ways to perform dental procedures, focusing on general dentistry. Dentists from all over the United States and Canada have traveled to Ripley to observe and learn his techniques and improve their own patient-delivery systems. In Dr. Griffin's opinion, greater efficiency allows the general dentist to produce more dentistry and take more time off. One of his greatest joys in life is spending time with his wife and three children, and he wants all dentists to have the freedom to spend as much time as possible with their families.

Dr. Griffin's many extracurricular activities include the charity, Dentistry With a Heart, coaching and sponsoring multiple little league sports, and serving as an officer in the Mississippi Academy of General Dentistry. In 2010, Dr. Griffin was honored with the Humanitarian of the Year Award by his peers at the Mississippi Dental Association for his community and charitable efforts.

Dr. Griffin still practices solo in Ripley, and can be reached at: chrisgriffin@thecapacityacademy.com.

CHAPTER 2

SLEEP APNEA: THE 'NOT SO SILENT' KILLER

BY JESSE CHAI, DDS

Imagine being 43 years old having had a 15-year career as a Professional Football Player in the NFL (National Football League) as a Defensive end. In fact you were one of the greatest and most decorated players in NFL history winning two NFL Defensive Player of the Year awards, 13-time Pro Bowl and 12-time All-Pro Selections and you help lead your team to victory at Super Bowl XXXI. You were the most feared Defensive Lineman in history. You were one of the top athletes in the world. Now, just 4 years after retirement at the young age of 43, you're dead.

The NFL Hall of Famer that this sad story depicts is of Reggie White, nicknamed "The Minister of Defense." Reggie White died December 26th, 2004 leaving behind his wife and two children. According to Keith Johnson, spokesman for the White family regarding Reggie's death, "A 43 year old is not supposed to die in his sleep. It was not only unexpected, but it was also a complete surprise. Reggie wasn't a sick man... he was vibrant. He had lots and lots of energy, lots of passion."

Having to deal with the death of your husband and father at such a young age is hard enough to swallow as is, but to lose him the day after Christmas will likely be hard for any family to cope with.

So what caused the death of this Once-Great athlete?

According to Reggie's wife Sara, Reggie had Sleep Apnea and was treated with the conventional CPAP (Continuous Positive Airway Pressure) machine, which consists of a facemask that delivers oxygen to the patient during the night while you sleep. Unfortunately, according to Sara, "Reggie was unable to wear the facemask because he was claustrophobic." Although CPAP machines have an almost 100% success rate when worn, many patients (up to 87% in some studies) are unable to wear it. So what could have been done to prevent Reggie's death?

The number one alternative treatment to the facemask for patients that cannot wear the mask is a dentist-made Oral appliance. The Oral appliance is also recommended by the American Academy of Sleep Medicine as the first-line treatment for mild to moderate obstructive sleep apnea. "If Reggie would have known about oral appliances, he might still be alive today," says Sara White.

This is one of the saddest stories I have ever heard of. Reggie's death was likely preventable if he had known about Oral appliances that treat sleep apnea. It is not like he didn't have the financial ability to have one made or that he was undiagnosed with the condition of sleep apnea. He knew he had sleep apnea. He just couldn't wear the facemask that was prescribed for him, and he was not made aware of the alternatives to treatment, which included an Oral appliance.

SO WHAT IS SLEEP APNEA?

There are actually two types of sleep apnea. One is called Central Sleep Apnea, which is a neurological disorder and occurs when the brain fails to send the appropriate signals to the muscles that start your breathing. It is extremely rare thankfully, and is not something a dentist would treat. The other type is Obstructive sleep apnea, which is much more common and for the purposes of this chapter, when I refer to sleep apnea, I'm referring to Obstructive sleep apnea.

Sleep Apnea is a serious, potentially life-threatening condition that poor Reggie White and many others have succumbed to, including Jerry Garcia of the Grateful Dead, who died in 1995 at the age of 53. It is widely suspected that undiagnosed sleep apnea contributed to the early death of the famous comedian, John Candy, who died in his sleep in 1994 at the age of 43. Sleep Apnea occurs when the soft tissue in the back of your throat collapses, causing a blockage which impairs your ability to breathe in air. With Sleep apnea, your breathing actually stops for 10 seconds or longer (sometimes up to **two minutes!**), and this can frequently happen hundreds of times per night.

Imagine being CHOKED for 10 seconds or more at a time, hundreds of times in one night... you'd probably feel pretty beat up and exhausted. Imagine this being your life every night. That is what happens when you have sleep apnea. You are basically sleep deprived for everyday of your life, which is a form of torture in itself. It is no wonder why they say that, left untreated, Sleep Apnea takes an average of **eight to ten years off a person's life!**

Now the scary thing is that because sleep apnea is so poorly understood and the awareness of sleep apnea in the general public is so poor, less than 10% of people that suffer from Sleep Apnea have been properly diagnosed or treated! In the US and Canada alone there are millions of people walking around undiagnosed with this life threatening condition!

SO WHO ELSE HAS SLEEP APNEA?

If you have sleep apnea, you are not alone. The good news is, the awareness of sleep apnea is improving and many celebrities have stepped forward to increase public awareness about their disease. Basketball legend Shaquille O'Neil, William Shatner (Star Trek's Captain James T Kirk), and Talk Show hosts Regis Philbin and Rosie O'Donnell all have sleep apnea, with the big difference being, they have been diagnosed and are being treated.

Isn't it nice to know that if you have sleep apnea you can still live a long comfortable life if you seek treatment?

Dangers of Undiagnosed or Untreated Sleep Apnea

When left untreated, Sleep apnea can lead to some pretty serious consequences including:

- Increased risk of heart problems and stroke
- Increased risk of high blood pressure
- Motor vehicle accidents or accidents at work
- DEATH

In other words, if you are at risk of sleep apnea or know you have it, you would be pretty foolish not to get it treated, wouldn't you?

HOW DO I KNOW IF I HAVE IT?

So by now, I hope you are at least asking yourself this question. As of now the gold standard is to go for an Overnight Sleep Study in a sleep clinic. The idea of sleeping in a foreign bed being monitored while you sleep may not sound like fun. However, if it will add eight to ten years to my life and improve the quality of my life, I think I can endure one inconvenient sleepover. Home sleep tests do exist, which are much less intrusive, but a physician must diagnose the results and they may not be acceptable for diagnosis depending on where you live. So before you go to your doctor to ask them to send you for a sleep study, we need to see if you have any signs and symptoms of Sleep Apnea.

SIGNS AND SYMPTOMS OF SLEEP APNEA

1. **Frequent stoppage of breathing** during sleep, which your partner may notice when you sleep, is a telltale

sign. If this is happening, you need to go see your doctor immediately!

2. **Choking, gasping or gagging** during sleep to get air into your lungs. Another telltale sign.

3. **Loud snoring** happens to be the **most obvious symptom of sleep apnea**. The problem is that snoring is seen by most people, including physicians, as an annoyance or a joke, or even a sign of good sleep. The fact is that snoring is caused by a partial obstruction of your airway, and even a partial obstruction in your breathing is not good. The combination of snoring, stoppage of breathing and choking and gasping for air causes very fragmented and poor sleep.

4. **Feeling unrefreshed in the morning** - imagine sleeping for 8 hours and still being tired... well, if you have sleep apnea and have interrupted sleep all night, it's no wonder you're still tired.

5. **Headaches** upon awakening. Oxygen deprivation can give you one nasty headache.

6. **Waking up sweating during the night.** I think I'd be sweaty too if I was being choked a few hundred times a night.

7. **Excessive daytime tiredness/sleepiness.** This is the most common symptom of Sleep Apnea and present almost 100% of the time. As a result, people with sleep apnea often have decreased performance at work, and mood changes. Sleep deprivation will do that to you. You are basically functioning impaired. The scary thing is, if you have untreated sleep apnea, you are **TWELVE times more likely to be in an automobile accident**.

8. **Lethargy -** lack of sleep will cause you to be drowsy, sluggish and have no energy.

9. **Rapid weight gain** - Your body is tired. You have no energy to exercise, so you are consuming more calories than you burn.

10. **Memory loss and learning difficulties** - Again, if you haven't had a good night's sleep in who knows how long, your ability to think clearly is next to nada. This applies to kids as well.

11. **Short attention span** - If you are beat tired, you can't concentrate.

12. **Poor judgment** - Sleep deprivation is not going to help you make very sound decisions.

13. **Depression** - If I haven't slept well in days, months, years, I'd be pretty depressed too.

14. **Personality changes** - Sleep deprivation screws up your brain chemistry. I know a lot of people that are grumpy only having one bad night's sleep (including myself)... imagine this going on everyday!

15. **High blood pressure/hypertension -** 60% of Sleep apnea patients have high blood pressure. If I choked you a few hundred times a night, the shock to your system alone will raise your blood pressure... and this is a nightly thing. So if you have High blood pressure, with no diagnosis as to why ... you might have sleep apnea.

16. **Acid reflux - GERD** (Gastroesophageal Reflux Disorder) is quite common in Sleep apnea. When your body is trying hard to take a breath, the negative pressure exerted by your stomach can cause stomach acid to come up. When treating sleep apnea, the Acid Reflux improves greatly and often is eliminated.

17. **Large neck circumference** - Unfortunately, if you have a big neck, there is an increased likelihood that you will have trouble breathing at night, as the fat in your neck and gravity restricts your breathing. Males with a 17 inch neck or greater, and females with a 16 inch neck or greater are at higher risk.

18. **Obesity** - Unfortunately obese patients are more likely to have narrow airways and thus have a harder time getting oxygen in when trying to sleep. I need to clarify that you do not need to be overweight or have a large neck to have sleep apnea, but having a large neck and being obese does not help.

19. **Large tonsils** - If you have enlarged tonsils, and I have seen some the size of golf balls, you will have a hard time breathing at night and your chances of having sleep apnea shoot through the roof. This is one of the main causes of sleep apnea in children by the way. (Yes, kids can have sleep apnea too.) So if you have really big tonsils, or your child does, you might want to get those out ... it's pretty controversial, and I know doctors don't like doing it these days, but oxygen and proper sleep are 'pretty darn' important.

20. **Allergies and mouth breathing** - Allergies and Sinus problems can make it difficult and sometimes impossible to breathe through your nose. The big problem is, that makes you a mouth breather. Mouth breathing irritates the tissues in your throat causing them to become red and inflamed. Mouth breathing also over time causes your mouth to under-develop, so you have a small mouth. A Small mouth and a normal size tongue is not a good combination as when you lie on your back, your tongue falls back, blocks your throat and you now have sleep apnea.

21. **Frequent urination/bed wetting -** If you have to wake up to go to the washroom a few times a night, or your child wets the bed... chances are you/they have sleep apnea. This is because when you get into deep sleep, your body produces a hormone that controls your bladder, so you can sleep all night and not have to go to the washroom.

22. **ADHD** (Attention Deficit Hyperactivity Disorder) **Symptoms** - This is especially true in kids as they get overactive and inattentive due to Sleep deprivation... in other words, they're wired. Adults can get that too.

23. **Nighttime awakening** - if you wake up frequently in the night, there's a really good chance you have sleep apnea. Choking hundreds of times of night will leave you a pretty light sleeper.

24. **Cyanosis** - this is when your skin turns blue from lack of oxygen. This can occur in extreme cases of sleep apnea.

If you or someone you know has any of the above symptoms, you might want to get assessed to see if you have sleep apnea.

TREATMENT FOR SLEEP APNEA

There are four main ways to treat Sleep Apnea:

1. **CPAP -** This is the facemask we discussed before that Reggie White could not wear. It works nearly 100% of the time if you wear it. The problem is it is cumbersome and noisy and compliance is awful (only 13% wear it).

2. **Surgery** - There are many surgeries that can be done to cut away tissue that is obstructing your breathing but this is often very painful, and the tissue often re-grows. In fact the only tissue surgery that I have seen work are when the tonsils and adenoids are removed,

but this almost always works best when accompanied by the next treatment option.

3. **Orthopedic/Orthodontic Treatment** - Orthopedic refers to bone movement, where a dentist can use appliances to develop and widen your jawbones. This not only creates more room for your teeth, but it improves your ability to breathe as well. With a small jaw, your nasal passages and sinus are narrowed and your ability to breath through your nose diminishes. By developing your upper jaw, the sinus and nasal breathing improves about 10% for every millimeter of development. Developing your jaws creates more room and reduces swelling and inflammation for the tissue in the back of your throat and creates more room for the tongue as well.

Orthodontics is often associated with Orthopedics so that we can straighten the teeth after the jaws are developed. The combination of jaw development and tooth movement through braces tends to yield excellent results in terms of health (improved breathing) and esthetics (a beautiful broad smile). Children with crowded teeth are excellent candidates for jaw development as we can create the space for their teeth so they do not have to have teeth removed, and we vastly improve their ability to breathe during their growing years. This is an excellent treatment for children that snore. Although you may think your child snoring is cute, it is actually quite dangerous. Children should not snore at all. If they do, they likely have sleep apnea. Fortunately jaw development will fix this.

With our modern diet and the processed foods we are exposed to, allergies, mouth breathing and poor jaw development are becoming more common. Fortunately, dentists can now help by developing your jaw bones to where nature intended them to be – which not only gives you a great smile, but the ability to breathe properly for the rest of your life. The best part is this can be done at any age, so if you have sleep apnea and have always wanted a beautiful smile, this might be the solution for you.

4. **Oral Appliance** - This is a dentist-prescribed appliance that, when made correctly, is extremely effective at treating sleep apnea. It has a very high compliance rate due to its small size. It is extremely portable, and much easier to transport when you are on vacation than a CPAP machine. Most of the oral appliances are designed to keep your lower jaw forward when you sleep, thus preventing your tongue from falling to the back of throat. This helps keep your breathing more patent and free from obstructions. As mentioned earlier, the Oral appliance is recommended by the American Association of Sleep Medicine as the First Treatment Option for Mild to Moderate sleep apnea and for those that cannot wear their CPAP. These appliances are also extremely effective at treating snoring for those that don't have sleep apnea, but have poor sleep (or those that cause their spouse to have poor sleep!).

Sleep apnea is a serious condition, and if you have any of the signs or symptoms listed above, you should get tested. Reggie White was taken away from his family too soon. Don't let this happen to you or your family. Getting diagnosed and getting the proper treatment could greatly improve your quality of life, and it might even save it.

About Dr. Jesse Chai

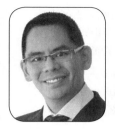

Jesse Chai, DDS graduated from the University of Toronto, Faculty of Dentistry in 1998. Early in his career he worked in nursing homes and around the Toronto area. It was in the nursing homes where Dr. Chai realized the true impact of improper dental care. After spending a year in Niagara Falls and Niagara-On-The-Lake, he eventually settled in Bradford, Ontario, Canada.

Dr. Jesse Chai is the owner and senior dentist at **Bradford Family Dentistry** and has been recognized for his contribution to the town of Bradford, having won the Entrepreneur of the Year award in 2006, the Customer Service Excellence Award in 2011 and the highest honour, the Business Excellence Award in both 2010 and 2012. According to the Bradford Board of Trade, this award is "presented to a business that has demonstrated outstanding characteristics in all areas such as performance, leadership, innovation, management, marketing and service." Dr. Chai is also very heavily involved with Community Sponsorships and Charity work. He hosts a Dentistry From the Heart event yearly, which is a free day of dental care for people in the community, and has donated over $31,000 in free dental care over the first two years of hosting this event.

Dr. Jesse Chai enjoys running a family practice and provides most dental services in-house, ranging from routine tooth-coloured fillings and cleanings to services such as **root canals, wisdom teeth removal, implants, dentures, ceramic crowns and bridges, headache and TMJ treatment, snoring and sleep Apnea treatment, braces and orthodontic treatment for children and adults, cosmetic dentistry and veneers, and Sedation Dentistry.**

Dr. Chai has incorporated a great deal of technology into his practice to help improve the patient experience and provide more efficient and comprehensive care.

Some of the great technology Dr. Chai has incorporated includes:

- **Intra-oral cameras** and digital cameras to help patients see what is happening in their mouths.

- **Digital x-rays** to reduce the patient's radiation exposure and allows patients to see more easily what is occurring in their mouths as images can be blown up to the size of the computer screen.

- **In-office crown making machine called Cerec AC** – which allows patients to receive Porcelain crowns and fillings in one office visit which greatly cuts down on office visits and the patient's time away from work.

- **Laser technology** for more rapid tissue healing and gum tissue treatment.

- **Cavity-detecting laser called a Diagnodent** to help find cavities at their earliest stages.

- **Oral cancer screening device called a Velscope** to help detect oral cancer at the earliest stages.

- **Electric motors** to reduce drilling times in the mouth and **rapid-curing lights** that can harder your fillings in as little as one second which greatly reduces your treatment time and the time you are in the dental chair!

Dr. Chai is married and has one young son who he enjoys hanging out with at home. Dr. Chai also enjoys reading, traveling and learning new things and is passionate about self-improvement. He can often be found listening to audio programs on his iPod, watching educational videos on his computer or traveling and attending live events. Dr. Chai enjoys watching TV and movies with his wife.

You can visit his website at: **www.BradfordFamilyDentist.ca**, or call the office toll-free at **1-855-DRTOOTH (378-6684).**

CHAPTER 3

THE MERCURY CONTROVERSY

BY DR. ADAM TAN, DMD, FAGD
DENTAL SURGEON

Mercury has a torrid history in dentistry. About 160 years ago, 'Silver Fillings' were introduced as a way to restore cavities and continues to be used by Traditional Dentists to this day. Attorney Charlie Brown[1] explains that the current use of the term "Silver Fillings" or "Dental Amalgam" is a misnomer. "Mercury Amalgam" better describes the material because these materials contain 50% mercury and a mix of other metals including silver (25%), zinc, tin, copper, etc.

Elemental mercury is considered the 2nd most toxic element after uranium. In dentistry, the controversy over mercury use revolves around how well mercury is 'locked' in Mercury Amalgams, and consequently, how harmless it is rendered within those Mercury Amalgams. Supporters of Traditional Dentistry believe Mercury Amalgams are safe. Anti-Mercury Amalgamists on the other hand, believe there is enough mercury released from Mercury Amalgams to make you very sick.[2] Members of each side of this debate are genuinely concerned. While Traditional Dentists and

1 http://bit.ly/ToxicTeeth
2 http:/bit.ly/Sfp9D4

Amalgam supporters wish that patients, especially those who are ill, will not be taken advantage of by unscrupulous practitioners, Anti-Mercury Amalgamists believe that all exposure to mercury in its various forms should be minimized, and if possible, avoided entirely.

In this chapter, I will convey the current view of the "Amalgam War" and hope you can review the links provided and make up your own mind. Presently, the overwhelming content in mass media is against the use of Mercury Amalgam in dentistry, and almost 50% of dentists are no longer placing Mercury Amalgams. In 1993, Dr. Hal Huggins wrote a notable book against mercury use in dentistry[3] but eventually lost his license.[4]

Those against the use of mercury in dentistry are vilifying mercury because they believe that the symptoms of mercury toxicity are insidious. The symptoms tend to be neurological and systemically degenerative, often mimicking other diseases. To the point that mercury toxicity due to mercury exposure from Mercury Amalgams has been implicated in Chronic Fatigue Syndrome, Multiple Sclerosis[5] (MS),[6] Autism, Alzheimer's Disease, diabetes, heart disease as well as acute symptoms such as hair loss, fatigue, fainting, memory loss, tremors and depression. The relationship to symptoms is from the predominance of mercury accumulation in specific organs, such as the brain, kidneys and liver.[7] There is evidence of changes in health complaints after removal of amalgam fillings, but the precise mechanisms remain to be identified.[8]

---

3 It's All In Your Head. The Link Between Mercury Amalgams and Illness. Dr. Hal Huggins.
Avery Publishing Group. New York. (1993)
4 http://bit.ly/HgToxicScam
5 http://bit.ly/MercuryMom
6 Multiple Sclerosis is a degenerative disease where the immune system attacksbrain cells,
specifically destroying the myelin sheath that insulates neurons.
7 http://bit.ly/VimySheepAmalgamStudy
8 http://1.usa.gov/OTecrm

Dental Governing bodies continue to discourage the indiscriminate removal of Mercury Amalgams. The Canadian Dental Association's (CDA) position as of February 2005 is that:

"Current scientific consensus supports the position that amalgam does not contribute to illness. There is no data to suggest that the removal of amalgam restorations should be performed in an attempt to treat patients with non-specific chronic complaints." [9]

The CDA stipulates that the patient must have a real, not perceived dental need, and has received sufficient information through a consent process.

If you decide to proceed with Amalgam Mercury replacement, there are typically five steps that are used by a Biological Dentist: Testing, Materials Biocompatibility, Getting Healthy First, a Mercury-Safe Removal Protocol and long term Lifestyle Improvement.

TESTING

You need to know the right test to perform, based on the suspected source of mercury toxicity. The test for chronic exposure – such as from diet and occupational exposure – will yield results with mercury blood concentration tests that can be requisitioned by your physician.

What most patients don't realize is that mercury vapor is released from dental amalgam fillings every time you chew – until they see a demonstration of the Smoking Tooth video from the International Association of Oral Medicine and Toxicology (IAOMT).[10] The average dose (3 to 3.5 micrograms per day) exceeds the *safe reference dose* (1 microgram/day) by at least 3 times to a maximal 8 to 9 times.[11] Dentists and patients can both assess if their exposure risk is significant based on Dr. Mark

---

9 http://bit.ly/CDAamalgamPosition
10 http://bit.ly/SmokingTooth
11 http://bit.ly/RichardsonHealthCanadaReport

Richardson's 1995 study of mercury risk exposure.[12] Some Anti-Mercury Amalgamists opine that there is no safe level of mercury, and any level of exposure is considered dangerous.[13]

BIOCOMPATIBILITY

Don't let the "cheap" price of Mercury Amalgams fool you. When you factor in the cost of environmental impact and long-term harmful effects to humans and wildlife, Mercury Amalgams are likely the most expensive dental filling material on the market. You do need to understand the risks: the act of removal and replacement of old Mercury Amalgams or any dental restoration with new a restoration (composite resins or ceramic onlays, etc.) can in themselves cause an inflammatory reaction from which the pulp of your tooth may not recover, resulting in the need for root canal therapy or extraction. Further, some Biological Dentists recommend that the dental materials must be assessed for biocompatibility to personally tailor a treatment designed for you. It can be a tremendous undertaking and you should proceed only after obtaining a sufficient and satisfactory explanation, and are comfortable to provide full consent.

GET HEALTHY

Get healthy before your proceed with the removal of mercury amalgams in your mouth to allow your body's detoxifying mechanisms to function normally and optimally. Certain protocols describe the use of supplements such as Coenzyme Q10 for the time leading up to the removal. Often times, a tincture is provided to the patient immediately before and after the removal process. These may include activated charcoal, chlorella and cilantro. Most importantly, if you are a female of childbearing potential, plan accordingly so that dental restorations, particularly the placement or removal of Mercury Amalgams, are not performed during pregnancy or when lactating.[14]

12 http://bit.ly/RichardsonHgParticulateDanger
13 Dr. Tom McGuire. Dental Wellness Institute. The poison in your teeth: Mercury Amalgam (Silver) Fillings…Hazardous to your Health! (2008)
14 http://1.usa.gov/TQSC69

SAFE MERCURY REMOVAL PROTOCOL

There are protocols that have been introduced by the IAOMT to reduce risk during Mercury Amalgam removal. Among them are:

1. Breathe an alternative air source provided through a nosepiece or nasal cannula. Don't breathe through your mouth during the procedure.

2. The tooth should be kept cool during the procedure to minimize mercury vapor production. Remember, heat application directly increases mercury vapor release.

3. Isolate the tooth. Do ensure that your dentist is using some form of tooth isolation to capture all of the old mercury amalgam during the removal process at the tooth site. A latex dental dam alone is an ineffective barrier against mercury vapor isolation, but can help to prevent swallowing the larger chunks of old Mercury Amalgam.

4. Chunking – the old mercury amalgam is cut using a technique that removes the old filling in larger chunks instead of smaller particles. Minimize the use of a diamond bur as it produces very fine dust that is difficult to contain.

5. Use a high–volume evacuator near the mouth to capture and filter mercury vapor, one that also ideally purifies the exhausted air through HEPA filters and a mercury-capturing filter substrate.

6. Thoroughly rinse the oral cavity after the removal process. In most cases a chelating or absorbing agent such as activated charcoal is used.

7. Dental personnel should wear protective gear, which may include canister filters that specifically filter out mercury vapor.

You should **not** allow a laser, prophy cup or air abrasion polishing to be used on the Mercury amalgam during the removal of old mercury filling – the heat and particulate generation, which is directly related to the amount of mercury vapor released, is difficult to contain.

LIFESTYLE IMPROVEMENT

Some Anti-Mercury Amalgamists recommend a regular detoxification regimen that includes chelation therapy if you have symptoms consistent with mercury toxification[15] and to only do this under the supervision of a physician or qualified medical professional. If a dentist provides chelation, this is seen as practicing outside of their field and is considered negligent in some jurisdictions.

A word of caution: There is currently no consistent regulation by the dental governing bodies on the designated terms that a dentist would use to describe the method of practice of mercury removal. Organizations such as the IAOMT are trying set standards that will help patients determine the level of training and awareness related to mercury sensitivity that a dentist has. The most common designations you will find are **Traditional Dentistry, Mercury-Free** and **Mercury-Safe.** Traditional dentistry practitioners incorporate the use of Mercury Amalgams in their practice. **Mercury- Free** dentists are those who no longer use Mercury Amalgams in their practice, but will necessarily still remove Mercury Amalgams. **Mercury-Safe** – typically refers to dentists who have implemented protocols to minimize mercury exposure to their patients, themselves and their staff, most specifically during the removal process of an old Mercury Amalgam Filling. In all cases, you should be provided with documentation, or ask to see additional credentialing, training or recognition from associations such as the IAOMT that have an accreditation process and in order to be satisfied that the dentist is practicing ethically.

---

15 http://bit.ly/MercuryChelation

THERE IS HOPE!

Most dental governing bodies support the use of the most appropriate dental materials for a particular condition. You have choices that can be used instead of Mercury Amalgams – including composites, glass ionomers and ceramics to name a few of the popular options. Your dentist should help you determine the appropriate type of material that is most compatible for you. For larger tooth restorations encompassing the replacement of a significant amount of tooth structure, I use a technology called CEREC. It's a treatment accelerator that helps me to create crowns, inlays and onlays using ceramics, all in one visit.

A final word: Consider your risk levels by finding out where your greatest source of mercury exposure is coming from and take the appropriate action. Are your exposure sources of mercury highest from your environment, your workplace or your diet? A diet high in certain predatory fish could be the culprit. Some cultural practices such as the emerging use of Traditional Chinese Medicine (TCM) in North America, have been implicated in higher mercury blood concentrations."[16]

Around your house, post-consumer waste containing mercury must be disposed of responsibly. Any mercury-containing waste from burnt out compact fluorescent bulbs, exhausted batteries or old broken thermostats, must be safely disposed of at hazardous waste sites to prevent mercury leaching into the environment. Here's what you can do at home: set aside plastic or cardboard containers to consolidate any hazardous waste in your garage or basement (provided they are still well contained, otherwise remove them from your home immediately!). Dispose of collected hazardous waste by bringing them to your community hazardous waste depot. Mercury waste that leaches from landfill sites will find its way into ground water, will then be taken up by bacteria that will convert elemental mercury to methyl mercury – the organic form of mercury that is readily taken up by liv-

---

16 http://www.ncbi.nlm.nih.gov/pubmed/1609495?dopt=Abstract

ing organisms. There can be a tremendous positive impact if we collectively prevent mercury entering into our waterways and oceans, and eventually back into the food chain.

As larger predators feed off hundreds of smaller organisms before them, toxins including mercury are concentrated in the predator. This process is known as bioaccumulation. The most significant of these larger predators are the fish we consume. The longer these fish are around (longer life span) the greater the amounts of bioaccumulation of toxins occur in their bodies. [16] Consequently, some of the largest fish from our oceans are laden with mercury. And guess what, as we consume portions of these large predatory fish – we are literally concentrating those toxins in our bodies as well.

Dr. Jane Hightower MD coined the term 'Fish Fog" for the symptoms resulting from diets containing a high proportion of predatory fish. Their symptoms include memory lapses, hair loss, fatigue, sleeplessness, tremors, headaches, muscle and joint pain, trouble thinking, gastrointestinal disturbances and an inability to do complex tasks. Limit your intake or eliminate consumption of freshwater fish and large predatory fish from the sea including Tuna, Swordfish and shark[17]. Demand mercury-free products to help reduce the amount of mercury reintroduced into our air, water and eventually entering into the food that we consume.[18] Coal-fired power plants have been implicated as one of the largest mercury polluters in the world – is that a big contributing factor that is affecting where you live? After looking at the available evidence, if you believe that your mercury exposure level is significantly contributed to by the Mercury Amalgam fillings you have in your mouth, and you believe they are affecting your health, seek help in formulating an opinion with your dentist, then decide on a plan of action on how you should proceed next.

17 Diagnosis: Mercury. Money, Politics & Poison. Island Press
  by Jane M. Hightower, MD. (2009)
18 http://bit.ly/MercuryandFishConsumption
19 Slow Death by Rubber Duck: How the Toxic Chemistry of Everyday Life Affects Our
  Health by Rick Smith, Bruce Lourie and Sarah Dopp (2009)

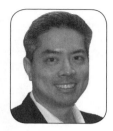

About Dr. Adam Tan

Dr. Adam Tan, DMD, FAGD is married to Wendy, whom he met at Queen's University in Kingston, Ontario, Canada, while obtaining his Bachelors of Science Degree with Honors. He went on to attain his degree in Doctor of Dental Medicine at the Boston University Goldman School of Dental Medicine in Boston, Massachusetts. Dr. Tan and Wendy are now blessed with three sons Ryan, Daniel and Lucas. Dr. Tan enjoys spending time and traveling with his family.

Dr. Tan's credentials include: Past President of the Muskoka-Simcoe Dental Society (MSDS), Fellow of the Academy of General Dentistry and Academy of Osseointegration, member of the Ontario Dental Association, International Association of Oral Medicine and Toxicology (IAOMT), American Dental Society of Anesthesiology, American Academy of Cranial Facial Pain (Canadian Chapter), American Academy of Facial Esthetics and the International Association of Orthodontics.

Dr. Tan actively promotes giving back to the community through annual dental charity events, providing Dentistry from The Heart events, providing free dentistry for all underserved members of the community. He participates annually as a major sponsor, fundraising for The Orillia Soldiers Memorial Hospital and the Ontario Provincial Police bike giveaways for their D.A.R.E programs in Barrie that promotes drug awareness for High School students and Children's Safety Village in Orillia which teaches public school children about traffic safety.

Dr. Tan has appeared on CTV News, the CBC Morning Show, KCIX and the Dock, Sunshine 89.1 FM Radio as well as several news articles in *The Orillia Packet and Times* newspaper.

His certifications include: Advanced Cardiac Life Support, Therapeutic Botox, surgical and prosthetic implant procedures, conscious sedation (oral, nitrous, and intravenous), orthodontics, Invisalign (he is an Invisalign Teen provider and recognized as a Preferred Invisalign Provider), and all wavelengths of dental lasers.

CHAPTER 4

THE POWER OF YOUR SMILE

BY AUDREY SIM, DDS

A woman came to me for an emergency visit with her crowned front tooth broken off at the gum line. The tooth could not be repaired and needed to be extracted. Thankfully the nerve had been removed when the original work was done so she was not in any pain, physically at least. Mentally she was distraught. The anguish of losing her front tooth had caused her to leave work early that day and she said all morning her coworkers were commenting on how she just wasn't acting like her usual bubbly self. Even the mail carrier who stopped in asked her if anything was wrong. She said she hadn't smiled all morning and had barely spoken to anyone which just wasn't like her. I assured her that we could give her a tooth that day. We could prepare the side teeth for a bridge and make a temporary bridge for her giving her a tooth where she no longer had one. She could then go at her convenience to get the root in the gum extracted. What happened next was nothing short of amazing. In my years of practicing dentistry I had never seen anything like what I was about to witness. My assistant and I prepared the teeth and fabricated the temporary bridge. When we handed her the mirror and she saw her old self again, not only did her face light up with delight but her entire body lit up from within as she returned to her bubbly self. She started talking a-mile-a-minute, making large hand gestures as she spoke, laughing using her whole body and smiling from ear to ear. She was a totally different person than the one who had walked into my office just an hour before.

The power of your smile is tremendous. It is an influential, key part of not only your appearance but your personal presentation and your mental health. You use your smile to convey happiness to your significant other, approval and love to your children, support to a friend, and appreciation to a co-worker. But it also is part of how you see yourself. Inside your mind's eye you have an idea what your smile should look like and you use your smile to reveal yourself to others about how you feel and what you are thinking. It is an important tool to communicate with the people in your life. So when you look in the mirror if the smile you expect to see or the smile you would like to see isn't looking back at you, it can be stressful and unsettling. And if you give up smiling altogether or cover your smile when you speak or laugh, you are hindering the social connection you have with others and bad habits can form that can have a lasting impact on our life. You may not smile at anyone and this can go on for *years*. You may cover your mouth when you laugh but then when your hands are full of groceries and you run into a friend outside the supermarket you can't greet them with your smile or laugh at their joke. Everyday you could be sending unfriendly signals to others, signals you don't mean to send. The effects of a broken smile can have significant and long lasting effects on your quality of life and these problems can keep you from moving forward and leading the life you would like to have.

Here are some powerful reasons to smile:

1. A smile makes you look more attractive because it draws people to you.

2. People who smile are perceived to be more competent and successful than someone who does not smile (so it really could get you that job).

3. Smiles are contagious. When one person smiles at another, ours brains are hardwired to smile back. We can't help it!

4. Smiling relieves stress.

5. People who smile wide and often live 7-10 years longer than those who don't.

6. Smiling boosts the immune system. It releases endorphins, natural pain killers and serotonin, the body's "happy hormone."

7. Smiling lowers your blood pressure.

8. Smiling makes you look younger because it lifts the face.

9. Returning a smile actually helps you interpret the other person's intentions more accurately. It assists your brain in determining if the other person's smile is genuine.

10. Even if you're sad, smiling can have a reverse effect and actually trigger the mind to feel happy. Think of something positive that will make you smile so your eyes smile with your mouth to get the full benefit.

As you can see, smiling is an important part of the social connection we have with others and is an important part of our mental and physical health. Are your dental problems keeping you from smiling?

THE POWER OF COSMETIC DENTISTRY

Cosmetic dentistry can provide wonderful answers to your smile problems. Many patients think of cosmetic dentistry as crowns or veneers and having to spending many thousands of dollars. But cosmetic dentistry can be as simple as finally getting that tooth bonded which you chipped as a kid. This procedure may only cost you a few hundred dollars or even less with the help of dental insurance. Whitening has also become more afford-able, and dentists and whitening spas often run specials. If these simple procedures will give you the confidence to smile your fullest, think about the return on investment!

Cosmetic dentistry includes a wide variety of services from simple bonding of a tooth to full mouth smile design and also offers multiple ways to solve a single problem. But don't let yourself get overwhelmed by the unknown and let the unknown keep you from seeking treatment. Don't worry about how you will solve your cosmetic problem – that is the dentist's job. Find a dentist you are comfortable with, tell them how you want your smile to look, and let them show you what cosmetic dentistry can do for you.

HOW TO GET STARTED

Start by visiting your general dentist, present them with your cosmetic concerns and find out how they would fix your problem. Many general dentists do cosmetic dentistry and have lots of experience but don't advertise as a cosmetic dentist or promote it in their practice. They may do cosmetic cases frequently and have the happy patients to prove it! Call for a consultation and hear what they have to say. They may have many cosmetic procedures in their tool belt. If you are comfortable with their answers and fees, then you need look no further.

If after seeing your general dentist, however, you want to keep looking, don't be afraid to ask them for a referral. Dentists know other dentists and know who is good and who specializes in various procedures. It will give you a better place to start than if you walk out of their office left to find someone on your own. A good dentist will respect your right for a second opinion and support you. But if you are not comfortable asking, great referral sources you can contact are the current president of your county dental society. You can find their name at http://www.ada.org/localorganizations.aspx (just fill in your state and county) or by contacting the American Academy of Cosmetic Dentistry at www.aacd.com. They can refer you to a dentist in your area who does cosmetic procedures.

YOUR COSMETIC CONSULTATION

Once you have some names of cosmetic dentists in your area, call and ask for a cosmetic consultation. Some dentists may provide this at no charge, some may charge a consultation fee while others may charge a fee and apply it to future treatment. Be sure to ask if there is a fee so you are not surprised. Tell the receptionist that you looking for someone specifically to perform some cosmetic procedures. This way you can avoid being scheduled for a routine check up or cleaning and the doctor will have scheduled enough time to speak with you.

Here is a checklist of things to think about; things to bring to your cosmetic consultation and questions to ask your prospective cosmetic dentist:

1. First, if you have a deadline for achieving your new smile, go for your consultation as soon as possible and inform the dentist. This may affect whether or not your dentist can complete your case in time. Cosmetic dentistry can rarely be done in one visit. The more complex your case the more time it may take. Give yourself time to fit your appointments in your busy schedule and allow time for lab work, critiquing, adjustments, and healing. Begin with the end in mind.

2. Think about why you are seeking cosmetic treatment and the goal of the changes you want to make. A clearly-stated goal can help your dentist make sure you are satisfied with the result.

3. Think about the color you would like your teeth to be. I have found every patient has different thoughts about this. Some patients want very white teeth while

others want a more natural tooth color. Your dentist has a guide of a wide variety of shades for you to choose from. Ask for a shade assessment at your visit.

4. Consider having a significant other, family member or friend to be your support person throughout the process. Preferably someone your own age or older or perhaps an adult child. Bring them to your consultation to help you stay on track especially if walking into a dental office makes you uneasy. Also ask them to take notes for you. This should be someone who you trust. Avoid choosing someone who is a naysayer in your life and avoid those people in general during the process. Reach out only to those who will be supportive while you are a "work in progress." I have also found that younger children and grandchildren can be harsh critics and their opinion should be taken with a grain of salt. They may not be used to seeing you with different teeth and if it is disturbing to them, they won't say so, they will just disapprove and may even be unkind. If this happens, it's best not to consider their opinions.

5. Bring a copy of your most recent x-rays to see if you can avoid having more taken. This may not be possible but worth a try.

6. Bring any photos of smiles you like or pictures of you when you had a smile you enjoyed. A picture, as they say, is worth a thousand words and can communicate what result you would like to see. A smile catalog is available at http://www.smilepix.com/lvi/index.html for ideas on smile design.

7. Ask the prospective dentist how long have they been practicing, how many cosmetic cases have they done, and if those patients were happy.

8. Ask for patient referrals and/or before and after pictures of cases they have done.

9. Ask what materials will be used, why they are choosing those materials and if there are alternatives.

10. Tell your dentist if you are a grinder or clencher, this may influence what materials will be used and if you will need to have a bite guard made to protect your new smile.

11. There are often multiple ways to solve one cosmetic problem. Ask to be presented with all the alternatives to solve your problem, and the pros and cons of each alternative.

12. It is the dentist's job to handle the technical aspects of your case and give you what you want. But sometimes the dentist is limited by factors such as your head and neck anatomy, your bite, your medical history or other dental work present in your mouth, and may not be able to solve your cosmetic problem in the way you would like. If they can't give you what you want, ask for an explanation so you can compare this with treatment choices you may receive at other consultations.

13. Ask if you can get a "wax up" or mock up of your new smile to see how it will look. There will be a charge for this that the dentist should apply to your case if you seek treatment with him or her so you may wish to do this once you have chosen the dentist who will do the work.

14. If applicable, ask to make sure you are allowed to approve the temporary phase of your cosmetic procedure. The temporary phase is a great chance to make sure you are getting exactly what you want and make changes before the final restorations are made.

15. Finally, the current state of your oral health can affect the outcome of a cosmetic case. If your dentist feels other work needs to be performed such as gum work before cosmetic restorations can be placed, ask for an explanation. If you haven't been to the dentist in awhile, you may need to reach a certain minimum level of oral health to achieve a successful outcome and ensure your new cosmetic work will last.

I cannot stress enough how one of the most important things about receiving cosmetic dentistry is for you to feel comfortable enough with your dentist that you can talk candidly with him or her. Effective communication is one of the most important parts of treatment success. You need to be able to communicate what you want to your dentist and be reassured they are listening. If you don't feel you can communicate with the dentist, how can you be assured you are going to get what you want? It is very important that you share your reason for having cosmetic dentistry done and how you want your new smile to look, because if you don't, your dentist will make these decisions for you!

For me the most exciting part of the journey is this first step, the cosmetic consultation, because I get to hear the story that brought the patient to this point. When I ask my patients why they want cosmetic treatment I have never been given the answer, "Well, I want to be look beautiful" or "I want to look like a movie star." Instead, I hear a story that is deeply personal. Each story is as unique as each patient and I feel privileged to know those stories and be part of them. One patient was certain if he whitened his teeth he would get a job (and he did!). One patient said he had not smiled in years and could not live that way anymore. Another patient, after a long divorce, wanted to enter the dating scene again and knew he needed a better smile to increase his odds (and it did!). One patient was a singer and wanted to look good for her performances when she opened her mouth. Another had a 20-year high school reunion, and another an important wedding. One patient always knew she had a bright, white smile inside her but could never get her teeth white enough to match the vision she had in her mind. Another patient had dark staining in her teeth from antibiotics as a child, and it bothered her all her life. And the list goes on.

I love the conversation that follows where the patient and I work together to plan their treatment. This means taking what I know about smile design and applying it to what the patient wants, and designing their own unique smile. That's where the power of cosmetic dentistry merges with the power of the patient's smile. Then at the "reveal" when the patient sees the final result, I don't just see the patient with their new smile, but I see a smile that comes from inside of them because they know their actual smile matches the one in their mind's eye.

Your smile is too important to your well being and quality of life not to have the smile you want. I have seen cosmetic dentistry enhance the lives of too many patients not to believe what a powerful impact it can have on your life too. Even if you are unsure if you want to seek treatment, I urge you to find out what options are available to you. Take that first step and schedule your consultation today.

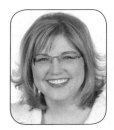

About Dr. Audrey Sim

Audrey Sim, DDS attended the University of Illinois at Urbana-Champaign, receiving a Bachelor of Science degree in Microbiology in 1989. She had intended to go into scientific research but discovered that in the practice of dentistry she could combine her love of science, her creative abilities and her passion for serving others.

Dr. Audrey attended the University of Illinois at Chicago, College of Dentistry, graduating in 1993. She then moved back to Algonquin, her hometown, and has been serving the people of the Northern Illinois Fox River Valley ever since. In 1995, she co-founded a group practice that was nationally awarded "Dental Practice of the Year" by *Dental Economics* magazine and the Levin Group in 1998 and locally awarded Best of the Fox, Best Dentist in McHenry County by readers of the *Northwest Herald* in 2003.

In 2008, she left her group practice to start her own solo practice, All Smiles By Dr. Audrey. Dr. Audrey provides general dentistry, cosmetic dentistry and same-day dentistry to patients of all ages. Her practice uses the latest in dental technology including digital radiography, lasers, and CAD-CAM, same-day restorations. In 2012, she was voted a *Top Dentist* by her peers in McHenry County in a *Chicago Tribune* survey.

Dr. Audrey is a member of the American Dental Association, the Illinois State Dental Society, the McHenry County Dental Society and the American Academy of Cosmetic Dentistry. She is actively involved in her community, annually sponsoring local events and providing free dentistry to newly-discharged, displaced and homeless veterans. She has been a featured speaker at the University of Illinois College of Dentistry.

Dr. Audrey also lives in Algonquin. She enjoys crafts, traveling, music, gardening, bird watching, digital photography, and spending time with her family and friends.

To learn more about Dr. Audrey and her practice, visit: www.draudrey.com.

CHAPTER 5

BETTER KISSES AND IMPROVED HEALTH: BENEFITS OF KEEPING THE TEETH YOU HAVE

BY BRETT SILVERMAN, DDS, MAGD

What do you think would happen if a tile or two broke or came loose from your shower wall? There are two ways you can address the problem; remove the couple of loose tiles, replace them and re-grout the area to seal out future damage, or remove the loose tiles and leave the hole in the wall and hope for the best. How much damage can really occur if you just remove the tiles and let the wallboard behind it fend for itself? …Plenty!

Within a short time, the wallboard behind the tiles will have absorbed water and allowed bacteria and mold to grow. The tiles surrounding the absent tiles no longer have protection from the elements and they can become loose and unstable as well. Ultimately the entire framework of 2 x 4's behind the scenes become part of the quagmire of mold and bacteria, thus causing structural problems that affect the health of your entire home in ways far greater than you might have imagined from the removal of a couple broken tiles.

So it goes with the removal of a broken or decaying tooth within your mouth.

It is tragic that the average person does not know or maybe does not want to know the link from oral health to systemic health. One might easily recognize the collateral damage that could be caused by the aforementioned missing tile in a shower wall, but not know the problems that a missing tooth can cause. Teeth are a critical link in overall health.

"If a person can take care of their teeth and gums, they can extend their life by at least 10 years," said Dr. Charles Mayo of the Mayo Clinic over 40 years ago. I agree with Dr. Mayo; I have witnessed it firsthand, but let me explain.

My grandfather had a very poor set of dentures that never seemed to fit him very well. It never was quite right; in fact, while I was in dental school he would ask if he could mail them to me and have me fix them. I would have to explain that I was still a student and I actually needed him to be present with his teeth in order to fix them. That I did not quite have my license, or an office, and that I could not just walk him into the dental school bypassing all the protocols established for patient visits did not matter to him. He understood and tried to act like it was no big deal, but my grandfather was disappointed that no one could help make his dentures fit better. He was unable to chew comfortably with his dentures. He developed a habit of taking a bite the best he could, mash it around a bit then swallow a large portion of half-chewed food, or as I called it, "The Big Gulp."

He obviously steered towards softer foods, but the process was the same: bite, mash, and then "the Big Gulp."

Near graduation, I received the call I knew would eventually come but didn't want so soon. My grandfather was in the hospital and he was going to die. The whole family from around the States flew in to spend a bit of time with him before he passed away. He was in the hospital for an inoperable bowel obstruction. Was my grandfather's death caused by his Big Gulp eating habit? I will never know, but as a dentist, I always have my suspicions. If you cannot chew and are swallowing hunks of food, I think it's a definite maybe. The tragedy was to watch him go from a sharp, with it guy, to someone who passed away within a couple of days knowing that there was nothing you could do and just sit by helplessly. We had to just sit and watch.

My grandfather's death reinforced my decision to pursue comprehensive dentistry. Do I think by having proper restorations, proper implants, or implant-supported dentures he would have been able to chew his food better and may have extended his life?

Yes, I do, as did Dr. Mayo. As dentists, we are the physicians of the mouth and often are the first to find health problems in patients. Overall health begins with proper nutrition; proper nutrition requires the ability to chew and properly digest appropriate and varied foods.

Think of all the things you do with your mouth in a day: eating, kissing, talking, or smiling.

What is a tooth worth...

- To a high school girl going to prom?
- To a man, who will smile as he walks his daughter down the aisle at her wedding?
- To the bride?
- To someone who is in pain and cannot experience the joys like other people?

My goal is to maintain people's teeth, their smile, and all the joys associated with their mouths. We can do better than what my grandfather had, and I fight daily to provide the best for my patients. Problems do arise, but how you handle them makes you who you are. We can fix that smile, we can replace that tooth, and we can bring joy back to the person who has lost it in these situations.

Sometimes the aggregate loss of a missing tooth is obvious as with a young girl who wants to smile with all her teeth at prom. Social standing may change when teeth are missing. Missing front teeth can keep one from getting a job or keep one from smiling so that one appears closed-off, unhappy, self-conscious, or unapproachable. However, missing teeth can cause a host of problems far less easy to recognize. Missing teeth can cause digestive issues. Digestion begins in the mouth with the chewing of food. Improperly chewed food cannot release the nutrients a body needs. Obviously, a missing tooth no longer does its job in chewing food, but that missing tooth also now puts the surrounding teeth under greater stress because the remaining teeth must work harder to grind food.

Chewing surfaces in the mouth still have to meet to chew the food, so the jaws may shift to allow teeth to align. Over time, the misalignment of the teeth may cause jaw issues and TMJ pain, as well as stress and strain on the ligaments used to move the jaw – which can radiate pain down the neck and upper spine. Aside from cosmetics or chewing, teeth provide structural support to the face. I describe the jaw as having two types of bone existing in your mouth, jawbone, and tooth bone. When teeth are lost, so are the structural supports in the mouth. No teeth no teeth bone.

One need only call up the vision of an elderly person with missing teeth whose face seems to have collapsed around their mouth to understand the significance of the support offered by teeth. Teeth have roots that keep the tooth bone and the jawbone. Removing a tooth creates a void where the tooth support no longer exists. What happens next is much the same as what happens in your yard if you remove a tree or bush and leave some of the roots below the surface—eventually, what was left of the roots decay and wither away leaving a soft hole into which the surrounding vegetation or even your foot might collapse.

Despite excellent oral hygiene, dental problems may still arise. When a tooth becomes damaged beyond repair, there are four options from which to choose for tooth replacement(and, yes, they can sometimes be combined):

- Remove the tooth and leave a space.

- Replace with removeable teeth such as a partial denture or a denture. Removeable teeth are the least expensive fix but they can move, do damage to other teeth and get food trapped beneath them.

- Bridge the teeth. A bridge involves filling the gap from a lost tooth by adjoining the teeth on either side to create a "bridge" of solid chewing surface.

- Single tooth implant. A single tooth implant creates a "fake root" for the tooth, thereby retaining the structural integrity in the mouth and mitigating damage to the surrounding teeth and jaw.

Dental implants can take a one-tooth problem and keep it a one-tooth problem. In the past if we lost a tooth, we would take that one tooth problem and convert it to a three-tooth problem by replacing that missing tooth with a bridge. If you have a small problem, why make it a bigger problem by including more teeth? With the greater dental options today, we can even address whole mouth problems with straightforward, implant dentistry. There are many different options available depending on the patient's wants, needs, and finances.

Are you motivated now to take charge of your overall health, add ten years to your life, AND improve your kissing by caring for your oral health? Follow these simple steps (with your dentist of course!) to decide:

What...your end result or goals are. A dentist should never assume, for example, that an elderly person does not need to have a pretty smile. Consult with your dentist, as I consult with my patients, to create a long-term goal for your teeth and mouth. If you notice something not quite right in your mouth--it doesn't have to be wrong nor does it have to hurt to be a problem--call a dentist to have yourself evaluated to make sure you're in the best oral health possible.

When...would you like to complete the process? Be up-front with your dentist. If you want to have a prettier smile for your daughter's wedding in a month, your pace to get the work done will accelerate. Patients frequently come to me with problems that have existed for a while, but that they wanted fixed...yesterday.

Where...will you get the work done? Choose your dentist carefully. There are great dentists around the country in all cities and small towns, you just have to call and make an appointment. If the office is dirty and cluttered, leave. It is always okay to leave a dental office in which you don't feel comfortable. If the dentist makes your feel uncomfortable, see another one. Ask a friend whose opinion you trust for a referral. Once you know what the issues are, create a plan to address it. In modern dentistry, we can handle just about any situation, any problem, whether cosmetic, functional or pain. The hardest part is just walking through the door.

How...will you achieve the results you desire? Excellent dental care requires a partnership. Your dentist should not do things "to" you, but should do things "with" you to improve your oral and overall health. For example, I will discern your comfort level by touching a shoulder or consulting with you during procedures. He or she will work with you to determine what dental insurance coverages you have and how to address your dental needs within the scope of your policy, addressing critical problems first and cosmetic fixes during an agreed-upon course of action.

When...should you begin changing your oral health? Today is not too soon. Nevertheless, let's be realistic. As anyone who has ever had to lose weight can attest, knowing that you need to do something is far different from being ready to do it! Emotions play a role in dentistry from the fear of pain to how a repair or implant will change our apprearance. Referring back to one's goal will keep each visit in perspective and keep the eye on the prize. In the words of French Philospoher, Henri Bergson, "The eye sees only what the mind is prepared to comprehend."

If you suspect we can change your life and health through dentistry...the answer is nearly always, yes. The overall health benefits of keeping all your teeth include better nutrition, healthier bone and jaw, fewer neck and upper back issues and improved social stature to name a few. Oh, and let's not forget...better kisses. They're important too.

All you have to do is make the first step, call and begin the process. The road to your destination begins with a single step. The choice is yours.

Are you going to make it?

Good luck on your journey. If I can be of assistance, please visit my website: www.SilvermanDentalCare.com and email me.

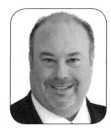

About Dr. Brett Silverman

Brett S. Silverman, DDS, MAGD, attended Eastern Michigan University in Ypsilanti, Michigan from 1989-1991 (Received early admission to dental school) and earned his DDS at the University of Detroit, Mercy Dental School, Detroit Michigan in 1995. He has the distinction of being the youngest member to complete the Masters Program in the Academy of General Dentistry (MAGD) in 2006.

He served as president of the NHL Team Dentist Association and served as chairperson of the NHL Athletic Mouthguard Committee.

Along with his partner, they were the official team dentists for the Atlanta Thrashers hockey team from their inaugural season in 1999 until their recent relocation to Winnipeg. He has served as an attending dentist for the SEC Football, Basketball and Gymnastics, member of the Board of Directors of the National Hockey League Team Dentist Association, as well as local youth sports. He has extensive training and experience treating traumatic injuries and their complex cosmetic rehabilitation.

He has been in private practice since 1996 in Duluth, Georgia as a general and cosmetic dentist with emphasis on implants and full-mouth-reconstruction cases. He has professional affiliations with American Dental Association, Georgia Dental Association, Alpha Omega Dental Fraternity, Academy for Sports Dentistry, NHL Team Dentist Association, NHL Team Physicians Association, and the American Academy of Dental Practice Administration.

Dr. Silverman currently resides in Alpharetta, Georgia with his wife, Hindy and their three children, Jonah, Joshua and Jamie.

To learn more about Dr. Silverman and his office, please visit his website at www.SilvermanDentalCare.com.

CHAPTER 6

CAN PERIODONTAL DISEASE INCREASE MY RISK OF A HEART ATTACK OR STROKE?

BY JIM S. CAUDILL, DMD

A STORY MORE COMMON THAN MOST PEOPLE THINK

They say the eye is the window into the soul.

Well, the mouth is the entranceway to so many ailments and afflictions, yet so many people ignore this serious fact. They go on living their life, worrying about trivial items, and ignore the need to see their dentist on a regular basis. I'm here to tell you that a dentist is not just responsible for your camera-ready smile, but also for your everyday health.

Dorothy was your average person, trying to brush her teeth everyday, floss occasionally, and rinse with mouthwash to strengthen her teeth and gums. She also went to see her local dentist the recommended two times a year.

Even with this apparent dedication to a healthy mouth, she

struggled with periodontal disease. We all know how frustrating it is in life to do the 'supposed' right things, but end up with less than satisfactory results. You feel trapped. You feel like there is nothing you can do. In the end, you want to quit!

Periodontal disease, also known as gum disease, is something that Dorothy could not ignore. Dorothy had read an article in a magazine that people with periodontal disease are twice as likely to have a stroke or heart attack as someone with healthy gums. Knowing the dangerous illnesses linked to this disease, she didn't have the luxury of just quitting without fixing the situation. With infected gums linked to heart disease, worsened diabetes, strokes and other ailments - she needed major help fast.

Needless to say, Dorothy was definitely not in Kansas anymore.

Luckily for Dorothy, whose real name I changed for this story, she came to see me after hearing about a new treatment with lasers. She had heard from trusted friends that this different and innovative method helped them with their inflamed gums, so she decided it was worth a try.

Our office happens to be one of the few dental offices in Kentucky that uses this revolutionary laser method against periodontal disease. Dorothy was desperate to see if these treatments could help her situation, especially after everything else had failed.

Having been in dentistry for more than 35 years, I've never seen results so positive for struggling patients – those who have tried other conventional methods with little or no success I told her this might be the solution she had been searching for all this time.

After doing a thorough exam on Dorothy, I diagnosed her condition as moderate gingivitis (infected gums) and moderate periodontal disease (loss of bone and other supporting structures around her teeth). During her exam, I noticed deposits of plaque along her gum line. Upon questioning her, I discovered that she was using a hard toothbrush and was shying away from her tender gums when brushing because of pain. I also found out that she was not flossing every day – which caused the gum infection and bone loss between her teeth.

WHAT LASER TREATMENTS DID FOR DOROTHY

When someone with periodontal disease hasn't had regular cleanings, the plaque around the gums becomes hardened and calcified. This might not be visible to the naked eye, but this hardened surface becomes a great hiding place for bacteria. They love to hunker down in the rough pockets and cause havoc on your gums.

The treatment I recommended for Dorothy was to have one of our hygienists thoroughly remove all of the calculus (calcified deposits), tartar and plaque from her teeth. This provides a clear pathway for one of our laser certified hygienists to do a laser treatment. Our hygienist uses the laser to eliminate diseased tissue and kill bacteria beneath the gums. This is a gentle treatment that can usually be performed without using any anesthetic. After two or three treatments I anticipated Dorothy's gums would stop bleeding and be much healthier. Once the gums become healthy, we frequently see bone begin to grow back in between the roots of the teeth, which is what I expected to see in Dorothy's case.

Now, the laser is not always a one-shot deal, and Dorothy had to come in for multiple treatments to kill the bacteria and get her gums healthy, but this is one of the more successful treatments I've seen in more than three decades in the profession. A cleaning does not always thoroughly attack the disease, so this new laser treatment might be the right method for you if you've tried everything else.

With Dorothy also thinking about starting a family in the near future, she was alarmed when I told her another result of periodontal disease was premature birth or low birth weight in babies of those suffering from the disease.

Dorothy's treatment went well and her gums no longer bleed when she brushes and flosses. Her teeth are stable and I anticipate her keeping them for the rest of her life as long as she continues keeping her teeth clean at home. She will also need to have her teeth professionally cleaned by one of our hygienists every three months to keep her periodontal disease under control and prevent other health problems.

I've always been skeptical of those stories where people break down and cry tears of joy after finally finding a way that works to heal a painful condition, but I watched first hand as Dorothy couldn't contain her relief. It was like all the hard work was actually worth it, and maybe she could live a normal life without pain in her mouth, bleeding gums and bad breath—or potentially worse problems.

Like with Dorothy, my goal here is to educate you and give you some potential signs of periodontal disease, as well as some tips to be proactive. This is one disease you don't want to procrastinate taking care of, and you want to be armed with all the information possible.

Periodontal disease is not something that just a handful of people deal with. It is extremely widespread, but most don't know they have it until it's too late. Chances are high that you or someone in your immediate family has periodontal disease. This is scary because this disease can be contagious. Don't use someone else's toothbrush. By the time a patient suspects they may have a gum disease and sees a dentist, the bone loss around their teeth may be so severe that laser treatments, gum surgery, or extracting some teeth might be their only course of action left.

Furthermore, it's usually not a very painful situation until you've had the disease for sometime – which is the scariest part. If you are one of those people that avoid the dentist like the plague, you might be in the thick of this disease before you even realize something is very wrong.

Think about it. Why do so many people ignore that when they brush their teeth, their gums bleed? If you washed your arm and it started bleeding, you wouldn't ignore that, would you? So if you have any signs of gum disease or have not seen a dentist within the last 12 months, get an exam as soon as possible. The main reason that I agreed to write this chapter is to sound the alarm that periodontal disease is serious and should be treated early. Failure to treat this disease can lead to an increased risk of a heart attack, a stroke, or make diabetes harder to control, as well as other health problems.

DON'T BE AFRAID – GO SEE THE DENTIST

There is a terrible stigma out there about going to see the dentist, but if you go regularly, it doesn't have to be a painful experience. Dentistry has come a long way in recent years as far as preventing pain during treatment. We have newer techniques and materials that make the dental visit more comfortable. We also offer nitrous oxide (laughing gas) which helps anxious patients relax. Nitrous Oxide also makes you feel less during treatment. It is important to get regular dental exams and have regular professional cleanings. By having your teeth cleaned by our hygienists and by keeping them clean at home, you can prevent periodontal disease.

If you have a diagnosis of periodontal disease, you should actually be going every three months, not just twice a year. You need more attention to keep the disease at bay.

Being proactive and getting regular cleanings can help soothe your pain and prevent further bone deterioration in your mouth. Don't wait until you see gaps between your teeth to decide it's time for a check- up. Remember, pain in your mouth means the disease is already advanced.

If you wait years to see your dentist, a mild case of gingivitis, that could have been treatable, can become the severe case we saw earlier with someone like Dorothy.

Plus, if you have been diagnosed with periodontal disease, it is something we can control and contain, but is not curable. This is a perennial disease, so regular visits to the dentist become essential. If you go beyond three months with this disease, statistics show bone loss can take place.

BE WISE TO THE CONNECTION BETWEEN YOUR TEETH AND YOUR BODY

The inflammation associated with gingivitis and periodontal disease has been determined to be a risk factor in patients similar to that of smoking as it relates to heart disease and strokes. Patients who already have other risk factors such as high blood pressure, high cholesterol or high triglycerides, obesity and family members with heart problems, should be especially concerned about keeping periodontal disease under control.

These are potentially fatal results, so think about that the next time you want to skip your dental checkup. Having periodontal disease does not mean that you will have a heart attack or stroke, but it can increase your risk of having one. Therefore don't take any unnecessary chances since periodontal disease can be prevented or controlled.

How does plaque form?

There is a biofilm that forms on the teeth every 24 hours. Bacteria in the mouth colonize or clump together on this biofilm. This forms a sticky substance filled with bacteria that we call plaque. The plaque feeds on sugars starches and carbohydrates. If the bacterial plaque is not cleaned off the teeth at least once every 24 hours, the bacteria produce toxins that damage the gums and teeth.

For further information, visit my website at:
www.hazarddentist.com.

SIGNS OF PERIODONTAL DISEASE

It is important to know what to look for if you think you might suffer from periodontal disease, which means scheduling an appointment with your dentist immediately.

Here are a few of the red flags to look out for:

- Swollen or tender gums when you brush and floss your teeth
- Bleeding gums, either when you are eating or brushing your teeth
- Pain when you eat cold or solid foods
- Shifting of the teeth
- Space between the teeth can mean there is major bone loss from the disease
- Loose teeth also means major bone loss
- Bad Breath
- Pus or bloody drainage when pressing on the gums

THINGS TO DO AT HOME THAT CAN KEEP PERIODONTAL DISEASE FROM GETTING WORSE

Home care can't cure the disease, and you shouldn't just do this without also seeing your dentist, but doing the right things in the comfort of your own home are essential to lessening the pains of periodontal disease.

Use a soft toothbrush, not a hard one. Many people believe a hard toothbrush is better for removing plaque. In fact, a stiff toothbrush coupled with a diagnosis of the disease will absolutely result in bleeding and pain. What happens next? The person becomes afraid to brush his or her teeth and shies away from the process, or doesn't do a good job of brushing around the gum line. So, use a soft toothbrush.

Make sure to brush along the gum line at a 45-degree angle to remove as much plaque as you can. Brush in short, circular motions, and make sure to only attack two or three teeth at a time. People often think they are brushing the right way, but brushing back and forth, while trying to clean as many teeth as possible is not the right way. Take your time, use the circular motion, and make sure to get the area clean in the most affective way possible.

Also, make sure to brush along the gum line on the inside portion of the teeth. There is a salivary gland under the tongue that dumps calcium there, so you must make sure to clean both the front and back of your teeth.

An electric toothbrush can often do a better and more efficient job at breaking up plaque than just using your average brush by hand. Whether it's a Phillips Sonicare or an Oral B Triumph, upgrade from the manual brush you might be used to.

Use an antibacterial mouthwash like Listerine or Crest Pro Health to further kill bacteria that cause Gingivitis. Rinsing the mouth for at least 30 seconds after brushing and flossing can reach little spots in between the teeth that brushing alone can't.

Make sure to floss daily and use the right technique. Use 18 inches of floss, and wrap the floss around two or three fingers for added tension and support. Use about one inch of floss in between the teeth and push it up around the gum line. Make sure to get the floss under the gums and around the teeth to break up the plaque that has formed. There shouldn't be bleeding when you floss unless you have inflammation. Bleeding should subside after about a week of proper brushing and flossing. Most people brush, but where we see the most bone loss is in the area in between the teeth from lack of flossing.

Remember your entire body's health and well-being is connected to your teeth in one way or another, so make sure not to skip any of these steps. Each is vital in its own way.

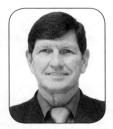

About Dr. Jim S. Caudill

Jim S. Caudill, DMD, PSC, has had a life-long relationship with the dental industry, getting his first taste of working alongside a professional dentist in high school. Jim always liked working with his hands and helping others, so it wouldn't surprise anyone who knows him that he has been in charge of his own practice in Hazard, KY since 1975.

The slogan on Jim's Website is "Cowards Love Us," as he prides himself on making patients feel comfortable and unafraid of checkups and dental treatment.

In addition to being in the dental field all his adult life, Jim is proud to be a resident of Kentucky for just as long, graduating from the prestigious University of Kentucky College of Dentistry in 1974.

Unlike most established doctors, Jim is never satisfied with the *status quo* and has taken post-graduate courses in numerous fields, including orthodontics, Lumineers, Invisalign, Implants, and periodontics – focusing on treating gum disease. He has added a new laser technique into his practice to treat gum disease, and is one of the few dentists in Kentucky to incorporate this new method.

One of the main reasons Jim decided to try the new laser treatment is his concern for his patients and helping people. The well-being of others is a top priority within his practice, so when he heard of the benefits that this new treatment could provide for periodontal disease, he jumped at the opportunity to give it a try.

"We've had patients that come in with bleeding gums, and they try the laser," he said. "The next time they come to us, their gums aren't bleeding anymore. So, we have had favorable reviews from the treatment."

For more information on Dr. Jim Caudill and his comforting staff, call 866-935-4005 or visit: www.hazarddentist.com.

CHAPTER 7

EXPERIENCE COMFORT IN YOUR DENTIST'S CHAIR

BY JOE GUROS, DDS

July, 1972, South Chicago Railroad Salvage Yard:
A yard foreman, Richard May, told me to tell "Jim," my co-laborer, that Jim would have to walk back to the yard office while Mr. May and I rode back in the truck. I told the foreman that I would rather walk back and that he could take Jim with him. He asked me why I was letting the black kid (but he used a derogatory word) ride, and I told Mr. May that I preferred not to hurt Jim as it was obvious that he, Mr. May, was being biased because I was white. He said a few nasty words, and as he drove off alone and shouted "Hell, I thought you were gonna be a dentist and they hurt people all the time with those damn shots."

As Jim and I walked back the mile and a half to the office," he asked me "Hey Joe, why do dentists hurt people with those shots all the time?" Not yet having taken a single dental school class, I told him that I didn't really know, but that I guessed that it was just the way that it had to be.

I clearly remember watching my older sister sitting in a dental chair and crying. The dentist came in and literally grabbed her head by her hair and pulled her head up so he could give her the "shot." I was only about five then, but that image is engrained in my memory. Events like this for a young patient can stay with them for a lifetime, and I'm pretty sure that Mr. May was remembering a similar experience.

Although seemingly a convoluted thought process, it did bug me for a long time and Mr. May's statement stays with me to this day. When I knew enough in dental school to ask about trying to give shots that were less painful, my instructors all seemed to agree that dental injections were painful and the faster that one could inject the liquid anesthetic, the better off the patient would be – having gotten it over with quickly. So I, as all of my fellow dental students, went through school administering local anesthetic in a fast, usually accurate, but always painful manner.

Graduating from dental school in 1975 allowed me to find an associate position at a group practice in Madison, Wisconsin. Our six-dentist office had me learning many things about dentistry that dental school could not teach. Of the many patient care procedures that this experience afforded me, the routine use of nitrous oxide analgesia/sedation is one that I carry with me today. Because my completing dental school accreditation early allowed me to attend post-doctoral education while still in dental school, I was able to learn about the uses of nitrous oxide in dentistry very early in my career. Dental school curriculum at the time did not provide this education, but I was fortunate to gain early experience with these post-doctoral classes. This class just touched on the proper use of nitrous oxide (N2O). My associateship in Madison allowed me to use it routinely.

N2O is a safe and effective adjunct to a comfortable dental experience for many dental patients, but unfortunately not all dental offices are equipped and trained to use it. Both of my subsequent dental offices that I equipped had N2O available in each treatment room. We rely on it to help some of our patients get through their appointment, and on the rare occasion that we run out, we feel somewhat lost without it.

N2O is but one part of our office protocol that we have developed to be able to give those "shots" painlessly on almost each occasion. Because some of our patients choose not to use N2O, we have developed over time other methods to aid us in obtaining that painless "shot." These methods are not some guarded secret that we choose to keep from other dental offices. On the contrary we wish that all dental offices would commit to these methods, so that the present and future generations can grow up without having the fear of dental injections that past generations have grown to accept as "that's just the way it is."

Here are only a few examples of what our extra care has given us:

A 20-year-old receptionist at our office was asked to fill in as an assistant for a few minutes. After observing me place anesthetic for her first time seeing it done, she later that day said to me "you know Dr. Guros, all these years when you would numb my mouth for filling work or taking out baby teeth, I had no idea that you were giving me shots. I can't believe that I never knew that."

A five-year-old little girl who we had treated with local anesthetic for some dental work returned to our office for a check up. She was behaving in a frightened manner when our dental hygienist asked her what made her act so frightened now – when she was never frightened in the past. She told our hygienist, and her mom confirmed this, that she was afraid that she was going to get a shot like she did at the other office. We had referred her to a pedodontist for retreatment of a failing pulpotomy (a type of nerve treatment on a baby tooth). The location of anesthetic given at the other office was the exact same area that we had given it but I suspect that it was done differently at the other office. After we reminded her that we do not give "shots" at our office, she calmed down and did fine thereafter. We do not want to lie to children, but end up doing so. We would much rather explain things when they are older.

A seven-year-old boy was at his second filling appointment with us when we noticed he was sitting back in
our chair with tears running down his cheeks. When we
asked him what was wrong, he told us that his friends
at school told him that they always give you shots for
fillings. It took a lot of explaining, reassurances, and re-
minding that we were just going to do the same thing
that we did the last time. After awhile, he was fine for
us to start treatment, however, it is a little more difficult to give a comfortable injection when our patient is
somewhat anticipating something will hurt. He did fine
though, and went on to brag to his friends that they were
wrong, according to his mom. He told them that he had
fillings put in with no shots!

Even though parents are good about following our request to not
mention shots to their kids before an appointment, it is impossible to stop children from talking amongst themselves about
dental visits.

We also have had many instances where our adult patients have
requested that we administer their local anesthetic before they
leave to go to a specialist's office for treatment (tooth extrac-
tions, gum surgery, root canals, for example). Having experienced our technique and that of some specialists, they have ap-
parently made the decision to allow us to administer their local
anesthetic for their treatment in the other offices. We detail for
the office that they are headed to exactly the type and amount
of anesthetic that we placed, and they can supplement it if they
need to. It is always painless to give anesthetic into an area that
is already numb, so any additional anesthetic that they place is
always painless. We do not advertise that we will do this, but we
certainly will help out our patients if they request it.

These methods have allowed our office to grow with the nicest,
most genuine, and oftentimes grateful patients that any office
could hope to serve. We are truly blessed with the best patients

that any office could hope for. These techniques have even resulted in patients returning to our office for their care after having gone to another office, because their insurance forced them to go there for better reimbursement. After comparing us to the often times assembly-line type treatment at PPO and HMO clinics, they tell us that they will gladly pay the few dollars difference to be able to get the care that we deliver.

This is not meant to be a slam against those types of clinics. They cannot help it. If they took the time and care that we do and then were forced to receive the compensation that some insurance contracts force them to accept, they could not stay in business with a profit. I firmly believe that our ability to take the extra time necessary to deliver comfortable treatment and our continued research into the latest developments in pain control have led to our attracting the very best patients.

This does not mean that other dental offices deliver sub-standard care or treatment. It simply means that many dental offices, due to insurance constraints, are unable to take the time and invest in materials and education to implement our methods. I also firmly believe that almost any dentist can deliver the same level of pain-free care that we do if he or she would take the time to learn these methods of care, and most importantly, take the time at the actual dental appointment to deliver care with compassion.

For our children patients, we will schedule first-time appointments that require anesthetic an entire half an hour over what we need to do treatment, so that we can slowly and carefully orient our new patient to all the new things he or she will be experiencing. We make certain that no injection will be noticed and then we proceed with the treatment. On subsequent visits we do not need to take as much time, because we have gained the trust of our little patients, but we still go slowly so as not to lose that trust. For our adult patients that already "know" what's coming at their first visit, we also take a little extra time to gain their trust, and subsequent visits start out much less stressful for them.

Our staff recognizes that our office starts out with a time-dis-advantage compared to dental offices that do not take the extra time necessary to make a dental appointment comfortable. This is what we mean. When office 'A' delivers anesthetic in a few seconds and not the ten to thirty minutes that we take, then office 'A' is more profitable for the same procedure. Although we charge a very small fee for local anesthetic, it by no means pays for the overhead expenses for the time used. There is no question that we lose money for a short period of time by the methods we use to make our patients comfortable, but I would not change what we are doing. It is rewarding to build a dental patient relationship that involves no fear of pain. These techniques are, as you will see, quite simple to incorporate but they do take time

Ten to twenty minutes or more per patient times four to eight patients a day results in our using one to two hours a day just administering anesthetic so that our patients are comfortable. Now we do use some of this time to do other procedures, but most of it is being right there with our patients slowly placing anesthetic with care and comfort. I know that many dentists reading this will think that we are foolish to "waste" this time but they are free to practice as they see fit. My point is that almost any dentist can do this if he or she is willing to take this time. I am not special in how I do some things, but I do take the time necessary to make our patients comfortable and if I can do it then almost any dentist can also do so. If a dentist is working at a pace that is meant to only produce as much revenue as possible, then this technique will not likely fit into their routine. It is also difficult to purchase the supplies needed if maximum profit is their goal.

So what is it that we do? I will break down our procedures so that anyone can follow what we do. One can take this to their dental office and request that they have their dental work using these procedures to help make their appointment more comfortable. Your dentist may not agree with what we do and I certainly would not tell another dentist how to practice. However this is what we do and it has worked very well for our office.

Our patient is escorted to the treatment room, seated and made comfortable with a super soft head pillow. After confirming the normal specifics of the appointment, topical anesthetic is placed on the area that will have the injection. Our topical anesthetic is formulated to our specifications through a pharmacy; it is not an average type as it is much more potent and costs more. I do realize that many dentists feel that topical anesthetic does not work but in our hands it does. We leave it in place for at least 90 seconds (if a dentist is in a hurry they will leave it on for only a few seconds and this will not work). If nitrous oxide is used, it is placed and our patient is allowed to breathe only oxygen for two to three minutes. This is done so that most of the nitrogen that is present in the air that we breathe is eliminated from our patient's circulation.

Nitrogen competes with nitrous oxide in our blood and its elimination results in a more complete effect of nitrous oxide. After a few minutes, nitrous oxide is gradually introduced to a level that our patient feels comfortable and relaxed. The topical anesthetic is removed and our patient's lip or cheek is gently held with a dry gauze square in the area to be anesthetized. A very small gauge (30 gauge) needle is used for this initial procedure. The area held by the gauze is gently but firmly shaken as the anesthetic is placed just barely in the tissue. Then, V-E-R-Y S-L-O-W-L-Y, just a few drops of anesthetic is deposited. I cannot overemphasize this step as slow and gentle EQUALS comfort. A dentist in a hurry will not be able to do this.

One of my dental assistants commented after observing me do this, "Dr. Guros, it seems as though the anesthetic plunger (which moves as the anesthetic is placed) stands still when you first inject, it hardly moves." And yes, that is how slowly it must move in order for a patient not to notice. After a minute, another very small amount of anesthetic is added. Then after another minute about one-half of a dose is placed. Then a minute later, the other half is given. A larger gauge (28 gauge) syringe tip is then used to safely place the final doses, so that precautionary

75

aspiration can take place just before the anesthetic is delivered. This takes time and if an office is under pressure to move fast to please the insurance, then this will not work.

Additionally, we have long ago invested in anesthetic carpule warmers. These devices gradually bring the temperature of the anesthetic to body temperature. The syringes themselves are also heated. Body temperature local anesthetic is less of a shock to the tissues as opposed to room temperature anesthetic.

We have always suspected that the acidity (pH) of anesthetic might also play a role in discomfort so we have routinely used a neutral pH anesthetic for the initial dose. This is another level of protection we provide against the sting of the shot. Within the last year and a half, we have invested in equipment that almost instantly changes the acidity of lidocaine HCl. This device requires yet more time, but it results in a body compatible pH so as to further lessen the possibility of anesthetic shock to the tissues. Most recently we have purchased a method to place anesthetic while taking advantage of the gate theory of pain transmission. Initial results are very promising where we will be able to place even the most uncomfortable injections in a pain free manner.

So the result is an anesthetic solution that is as close to the chemistry and temperature of our body tissues as possible and a method that is not perceptible as being uncomfortable. As one can see, these methods are not too difficult to incorporate if a dentist commits to taking the time to help patients.

If you think at all that another dentist could not do these things you are incorrect. I have trained our dental hygienists to do these same procedures, and when they take their time they obtain the very same painless shots. So I know that anyone trained and licensed to give local dental anesthetic can do this if they know the technique and invest to obtain the proper equipment and supplies. All of this costs more than the quick shot, but it is there to use if one wants to do so.

So dentists, take the time to help your patients; and patients, discuss this with your dentist if you would like to have a comfortable dental appointment. If the children presently seeing dentists for treatment experience complete comfort, then this whole generation can grow up without the fear that I and many others in my generation have engrained in their memory.

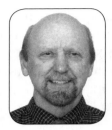

About Dr. Joe Guros

From working on weekends at 14 years of age unloading grocery trucks in East Chicago, Indiana, to railroad yard work in south Chicago, to working above the iron melting pots in Gary, Indiana's steel mills, Dr.Joe Guros, DDS had developed a strong work ethic and realized early on what an education can do for a person.

Making the switch from manual labor to intense study, he graduated from Purdue University in West Lafayette, Indiana in 1972 with a Bachelor of Science degree. Three years later he earned a Doctor of Dental Surgery degree with honors from Indiana University School of Dentistry in Indianapolis, Indiana. He was inducted into the OKU dental honor society while in dental school.

A self-described "dental nerd," he still spends most of his free time continuing his dental education. He feels that most dentists are good at their profession, but he knows that very few spend every free minute reading about new techniques and improving their patient care skills as he does. He is not one 'to toot his own horn' so to speak, so he has quietly, with the help of a fantastic staff, built a dental practice based on patient comfort.

His post graduate education includes: Functional Orthodontics, Invisalign Certification, membership in the International Association of Mini Dental Implant Dentists, Certification in Neuromuscular Occlusion, and countless dental seminars that earned him the Wisconsin Dental Association Continuing Education Award.

Most recently he became one of the first dentists to obtain Wisconsin state certification to administer Conscious Sedation enterally.

Dr. Joe's well-rounded exposure to many disciplines of dentistry allowed him to deliver patient care that focuses on comfort. He attributes having a dental practice with the nicest patients that any dentist could hope for to his well educated, dedicated, and professional staff. He has often stated that without their support, he would not have the passion and drive to sustain a top-notch office.

In this chapter he discusses some of the details of their painless dental practice, and challenges other dental offices to provide the most comfortable care possible for their patients.

Dr. Joe Guros maintains his office in Fort Atkinson, Wisconsin.
You can contact Dr. Guros at: 920-563-6373
Or at his web address: www.fortdentalcare.com

CHAPTER 8

ORTHODONTICS - NOT JUST FOR KIDS ANYMORE

BY BRIAN BERGH, DDS, MS

She walked through our door with apprehension, unsure of what might be in store for her that day. Somewhat shy, hesitant about being someplace where she thought only kids should go. Her friends all told her she was crazy to even think about it, even though both her adult daughter and 3 granddaughters had done the same thing years before.

Mary Jane, at age 72, was told that she was too old; that she shouldn't be so focused on herself; that a grandmother had better things to do with her time and money.

She'd recently had a discussion with her dentist. In that discussion she mentioned her concern about the way her upper front teeth looked. She wasn't really happy with how one particular tooth looked, and her dentist agreed that it could be changed.

Of the options available, Mary Jane's dentist, Dr. Turner, felt the best option was to align her teeth through orthodontic treatment first and then redo the crown that was done on that tooth many years ago. You see, her dentist felt that trying to redo only the crown to align her teeth would be the wrong choice. Even though it might be quicker, the long-term health and final result would be much better if her teeth were aligned first.

So that's what brought Mary Jane to our orthodontic office on that particular day – a suggestion from her dentist that orthodontic treatment would be the best long-term solution to a problem that had bothered her for years. This was a solution that would be in her best interest, giving her the best results and the best dental health possible.

These conversations are often difficult for both the patient and the dentist. And adults often don't even consider the thought of straightening their teeth, because they've been told by many, including their family, friends and even other dentists, that they shouldn't worry about their smile. They shouldn't be concerned about how they look. That they are fine just the way they are.

But as you and I both know, even as we get older, and maybe especially because we are getting older, our looks do still matter. A lot of things happen to our bodies as we age, things we never thought possible. So we start looking for ways to re-set the clock, to create a better us.

It's important that we continue to feel good about ourselves. Because how we feel about ourselves affects our quality of life and the way we interact with others, how we present ourselves and how we are perceived by others. This is not to mention that crooked teeth can also pose health problems – especially with the ability to keep our teeth clean and healthy. You see, as we get older, it's not unusual to experience some bone loss around the roots of the teeth. And teeth also move and shift as we age.

We are all familiar with the term osteoporosis and that our bones become more fragile as we get older. Think of the stories you've heard about elderly people falling and breaking a hip or leg. Well, the bone doesn't just go away from only those areas. It can also disappear from around the roots of the teeth, too. And when this happens, there is a greater chance of continued bone loss, especially when the teeth are crooked and can't be kept clean.

Crooked and mal-aligned teeth are likely to occur as we age. It's a natural process, but one that we don't need to accept as fate. Crooked and mal-aligned teeth can be fixed at any age.

Aldy, our oldest patient, is now 92 years old. He is a wonderful gentleman, who at the age of 86 decided he wanted to be proud of his smile once again. His orthodontic treatment took about a year to complete, and he still comes in to see us yearly to have his retainer checked.

Another patient, Jim, in his early 80's, wanted the same thing also - to be proud of his smile. One of the by-products of Jim's treatment was that he "felt like a kid again."

The average orthodontic practice has about one out of five patients over the age of 18. Eighteen is considered an adult in our field. Personally, I'm not convinced that a person should be called an adult any time before age twenty-five, maybe even forty. But, I digress. The point is that adults do seek orthodontic treatment and that number is continually increasing.

We have, in our office, been blessed with over one-third of our patients being adults. That's about 2 out of five, almost double the national average. Maybe this is the area in which my practice is located, but I think it's more due to embracing the idea of adult treatment, spending the extra time for additional education in adult treatment, and becoming an expert in the types of "braces" most popular to adults.

Most adults are skeptical of having braces bonded (glued) to their teeth like kids have. There is still a stigma attached to having the metal braces showing on the teeth. And although we've had some of our younger adults start getting "carded" at restaurants after having braces put on, older adults are not quite as excited about having the metal mouth look. Even clear braces with tooth-colored wires are not as popular with our adult patients.

That's why we've chosen to include the more cosmetic options of clear aligners (Invisalign in our office) or concealed, behind the teeth braces. Both of these orthodontic appliances are very cosmetic and hard to see. And that's what most adults desire these days.

In past years, a phenomenon in the dental field called "instant orthodontics" became popular. This was where the teeth could be "straightened" in two appointments. This often required a significant removal of the tooth enamel, sometimes to the point where a root canal was needed on one or more teeth.

Fortunately, this treatment has all but disappeared from the dental field as many dentists providing this type of treatment realized that it was not in their patient's best interest to straighten teeth this way. Not to mention, the results were often less than desirable due to problems matching the teeth to make them look normal and natural. That's why Mary Jane's dentist recommended orthodontic treatment before any dental work was completed.

Today's orthodontic treatment is different than it was years ago. I know when I had braces in the early 1970's, there was a lot of metal placed in the mouth. So much so that kids were often called "brace face" and the braces were referred to as "railroad tracks."

Through technology, orthodontic "braces" have changed to where even the metal braces are much less visible than before. With mini-brackets, tooth-colored brackets, and even tooth-colored wires, the braces are much less visible. And the best news is that now there are braces that are almost completely invisible when they're being worn!

The two most common "cosmetic" braces, or "invisible" braces are concealed braces, ones that are placed on the inside of the teeth by the tongue, and the clear removable aligners like Invisalign.

With these braces, adults can be confident that their braces won't outshine their personality and become the topic of conversation. That is, unless they want them to be. You see, many of our adult patients love to tell their friends and family about their orthodontic treatment and show off their new braces, which may not even be noticed.

One of my employees wanted Invisalign treatment. Being around the office and seeing the changes that our patients were going through, how much they appreciated their new smiles, how much more confident they felt about themselves, and how much more attractive they felt, she decided she wanted that, too.

So Susan, at age 47, committed to starting Invisalign treatment.

On the day her aligners were delivered she was excited. She could see, in her mind, the changes that were going to happen, and that she would feel more confident and proud of her smile, something she'd been thinking about for years. She was concerned, though, that her husband would notice and might make fun of her for trying. That she would be considered vain.

Well, her husband didn't say these things at all. In fact, after 3 days of wearing them, Susan had to show her husband that she was wearing the clear aligners. He hadn't even noticed that she'd been wearing them.

…And her girlfriends? Well, let's just say they were a bit envious of how attractive her new smile became. In fact, several of her friends decided to do the same thing. They became Invisalign patients, too.

So, how does one find out if they are a candidate for orthodontic or Invisalign treatment?

It's really quite easy.

The best orthodontic patients are people who have a dentist and see that dentist regularly. The overall health of the teeth, gums and bone surrounding the teeth should be good. Now, there can be some problems areas like those mentioned earlier due to crowding and mal-alignment of the teeth. We can't expect someone with crooked teeth to have perfectly healthy gums, because that's why treatment is often needed in the first place.

And you don't necessarily need a referral or recommendation from your dentist before calling for an orthodontic evaluation. Although, if your dentist does recommend an orthodontic evaluation, by all means follow their directions.

We have many patients who come to us directly with their concerns. They may not have even talked to their dentist about those concerns because they were never brought up during their regular dental appointments. In years past, orthodontic treatment was considered only for children and teenagers even by the dental profession. And many dentists do still carry that thought in their minds. So don't be afraid or concerned about seeking the advice and wisdom of an orthodontist even though your dentist hasn't mentioned you do so.

So how do you go about finding an orthodontist? Well, let me first explain a little about what an orthodontist is.

Orthodontists are dentists who have gone through significant additional training in the field of orthodontics and dento-facial orthopedics. This is a two-to-three-year <u>full time</u> program specifically associated with the training in the understanding of growth and development, orthodontic tooth movement, surgical orthodontic treatment and many other areas. The orthodontic program also includes a Master of Science degree in an area like craniofacial biology.

Why is this important to you?

In the dental profession, any dentist can perform orthodontic treatment. The training in dental school is generally very limited, often to only one or two classes during the entire four-year program. And a dental student may only treat one or two patients with orthodontic treatment.

An Orthodontist will have treated a hundred or so patients even before graduating from the specialty orthodontic program. They will have gained the knowledge and understanding to treat both easy orthodontic treatments all the way up to more complex treatments involving other dental specialists. This is important when treating adults, especially adults in their 40's, 50's, 60's, 70's and beyond. The understanding of how teeth move, the limitations of that tooth movement, and the response of the bone and gum tissue around the teeth is critical in creating a successful orthodontic treatment program.

The best place to start looking for an orthodontist is at the website: www.MyLifeMySmile.org. This website has been provided by the American Association of Orthodontists (AAO) and has a geographical listing of specially-trained orthodontists, those who have completed their specialty training through an accredited and approved program.

The next step would be to ask friends and neighbors, either adults or parents of children going through orthodontic treatment. See how they feel about the orthodontist they are seeing and whether they feel comfortable and confident recommending that doctor and that office.

Then, take the name or names of these doctors and compare them to the list you got from the website mentioned above. These are the orthodontists that you want to find more information about.

And if you're interested in the Invisalign clear aligners, there is one more step to take before calling and scheduling an orthodontic evaluation. This next step is to go to the Invisalign website at: www.Invisalign.com. At that site, you can find out how experienced the Orthodontist is in providing this type of treatment. Invisalign has been around since 1999, and there have been many advancements in the treatment over those years. You'd like to find someone who has the experience to take your situation and evaluate whether you are a candidate for Invisalign treatment.

On the Invisalign website, you can locate an Invisalign provider in your area. They can be found through a zip code directory on the site. Being close to your orthodontic office is important, but driving 5, 10, 15 or more miles to the right office might be the best choice you can make.

There are several levels of Invisalign experience. There is also a notation about whether the doctor is an Orthodontist or general dentist. As mentioned before, the value of seeking advice and treatment from an Orthodontist is that you can be sure this doctor has extensive training in the field of orthodontics and tooth movement.

Elite Preferred Invisalign doctors have the most experience treating with Invisalign. I recommend looking at these doctors first, especially if you have more than just a couple of millimeters of crowding. The Invisalign system has a unique way of aligning the teeth which is different from traditional braces. Those doctors with more experience will feel more comfortable and confident treating adult patients.

So, if you've been thinking about your smile, and deep down you'd love to be able to smile with confidence once again, what are you waiting for? The possibilities are endless in creating that beautiful smile you've been dreaming about. A little research, nothing too difficult, and a phone call to the right office will get you on your way to that beautiful and healthy smile.

Go ahead and schedule your appointment; most orthodontic offices will offer you a complimentary evaluation to let you know whether you are a candidate for orthodontic treatment. You'll also find out how long it will take and the investment you'll make to get that beautiful smile.

You deserve to feel good about yourself, again. Don't be afraid or nervous, find a qualified orthodontist who you can see, and make that appointment. It's never too late to have a beautiful and attractive smile.

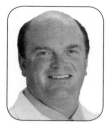

About Dr. Brian Bergh

Brian H. Bergh, DDS, MS is a 2nd generation orthodontist following in the footsteps of his father, Dr. Harold Bergh. Dr. Brian Bergh started in the orthodontic field at the tender young age of 13 working for his father as a lab technician. His love for orthodontics continued to grow as he continued to work in his father's office through high school and college. Dr. Bergh graduated from Loma Linda University Dental School in 1990, and served as president of his dental class for two years. He was elected to the OKU Dental Honor Fraternity, an honor reserved for the top 10% of dental students nationwide. Dr. Brian Bergh entered the University of Southern California graduate orthodontic program by invitation, and earned his Master of Science Degree in Craniofacial Biology and a Certificate in Orthodontics in 1992.

Dr. Bergh maintains an active role in his local community, as well as in the dental field. Dr. Bergh has served as President of the Glendale Academy of Dentists, the USC Orthodontic Alumni Association, and the Glendale Healthy Kids. He is currently the President of the Glendale Noon Rotary Club. Dr. Bergh also spent several years as a regional editor for the *Pacific Coast Society of Orthodontics Bulletin*. Dr. Bergh has served as a Clinical Professor at the USC School of Dentistry, where he's lectured and instructed dental students in Orthodontics. He currently holds study clubs instructing general dentists and dental hygienists about Orthodontics and Invisalign.

Dr. Bergh believes that education is the key to providing the best orthodontic treatment available. He routinely earns over 75 (3 times the required amount) hours of continuing education credits each year, with more than half of those hours concentrating on the Invisalign Treatment System.

Dr. Bergh has been recognized as one of America's Top Dentists for several years and was also voted Best Orthodontist in Glendale and the Foothill area many times. His office has received the Talk of the Town 5-star award for outstanding customer service for the 3 past years in a row.

Dr. Bergh is married to his lovely wife, Tina, who he met through the orthodontic profession. They have 3 children, Kaila, Kaigan and Bryley, a wild and spirited Poo-chon named Maddi and 4 Koi fish in their backyard pond. Dr. Bergh loves to go to Magic Mountain and ride the coasters, to Dave & Busters to play the video games, and to the movies to see the latest comedy films.

CHAPTER 9

A HEALTHY MOUTH AND BODY FROM THE START

BY FRANK ORLANDO, DDS, FAGD, FICOI

I recently went to the OB/GYN with my wife to discuss starting a family. The conversation centered on the importance of a healthy body and life style. My wife asked questions about exercise, what and what not to eat and on pre-natal vitamins. Like my wife, many women at this exciting stage in their life overlook the role oral health plays in their overall health.

For years the mouth has not really been considered part of the systemic body, and medical physicians and dentists have not teamed together to provide optimum oral systemic health. This is starting to change as more evidence emerges linking oral health to other parts of the body.

I have come across many situations where oral neglect leads to emergency dentistry at inopportune times. In the case of pregnancy, women who are trying to become pregnant should see their dentists as soon as possible to ensure their gums and teeth are completely healthy and bacteria free. Studies show that women with gum disease take, on average, two months longer to get pregnant than those who do not. Non-Caucasians with periodontal disease take, on average, 12 months longer to get pregnant. One simple appointment can save you months of trying.

Once pregnant, moms to be need to consider oral health in relation to:

- Pre-Term Birth
- Low Birth Weight
- Fetal Development

Finally, once baby arrives, mom will need to get up to speed on:

- Baby's oral health home care
- Teething
- First dental appointments

ORAL SYSTEMIC HEALTH

An expecting mother should have the goal to do whatever she can to provide the best possible environment for her unborn baby. We want to prevent pre-term birth and low birth weight and provide a healthy environment for optimal growth and health.

Newborns deserve the right to enter life with the best chance to thrive. This can be accomplished through the mother taking extra special care of her mouth and her body prior to giving birth, and continuing preventative and maintenance care throughout her life.

In 2001, the Surgeon General declared that periodontal health is of utmost importance and periodontal disease must be treated as a disease of the mouth as well as the body. In fact, it has been well documented that periodontal disease has been intimately linked to:

- Pre-Term Birth
- Low Birth Weight
- Fetal Development

And in general:

- Cardiovascular Disease
- Pulmonary Disease
- Diabetes
- Orthopedic Implant Failure
- Kidney Disease
- Pancreatic Cancer
- Oral Cancer
- Premature Death
- Erectile Dysfunction
- Rheumatoid Arthritis
- Alzheimer's Disease

PREGNANCY AND DENTAL WORK

Being pregnant is a very exciting time. Your body goes through multiple changes and new priorities take place. As a dentist, a valuable message I like to pass along is: **Don't neglect your dental health!** Recent research has found that maintaining oral hygiene can prevent many problems not only with a mother's health, but also with a baby's birth and health, including low birth weight and pre-term delivery.

PREGNANCY GINGIVITIS

The shocking truth is that **pregnancy gingivitis affects anywhere from 50 to 70 percent of pregnant women,** and those with the disease are **7 times more likely to go into preterm labor, preeclampsia, and have low-birth-weight babies!** Premature infants are at greater risk for short and long term complications, including disabilities and impediments in growth and mental development. Additionally, if an **expectant mom had untreated tooth decay and/or consumed a lot of sugar, their children have 4 times the risk of developing tooth decay!**

Ultimately, hormonal changes during pregnancy affect the body's natural response to dental plaque, which affect how gum tissues react to the bacteria in plaque; thus resulting in a higher chance of pregnant women getting gingivitis. Moreover, if you already have gingivitis going into a pregnancy, it will likely get worse during pregnancy if you do not seek treatment. Although gingivitis generally subsides shortly after birth, it should be periodically monitored by your dentist (during and after pregnancy), in order to prevent the gingivitis from turning into the more serious (and irreversible) form known as periodontitis.

To sum up, pregnancy gingivitis is a real and prevalent threat; but so long as you take the appropriate steps, it can be managed with relative ease.

The following are guidelines in response to the increased concern about oral health during pregnancy:

1. **Oral Health Education** – DO have consultations with your dentist before, during and after your pregnancy. Early intervention is key, but ongoing care is just as important!

2. **Oral Hygiene** – DO brush and floss regularly – and properly. It is especially important to try and always brush after meals and snacks, especially sugary ones. **Also, have more frequent dental cleanings than you normally would (2-3 during your pregnancy is about right).** This will greatly increase the amount of plaque that is removed from the teeth and gums, thereby lowering your risk.

3. **Nutrition** – DON'T eat junk food. This is good advice in general during your pregnancy, but just know that proper diet and nutrition during pregnancy will limit sugar intake, which, in turn, will minimize plaque build up.

4. **Treat Tooth Decay** – DO try and have all urgent dental

work completed prior to becoming pregnant. Although, it is safe to perform certain emergency dental procedures during your pregnancy, it is best to have it done prior to becoming pregnant, and especially prior to it becoming an emergency dental treatment!

5. <u>**Transmission of Bacteria**</u> – DON'T share food and utensils, so as not to potentially transmit bacteria known to cause tooth decay.

6. <u>**Use of Xylitol Gum**</u> – DO chew gum. Expectant mothers, and everyone, are encouraged to chew xylitol gum (around 4x/day), since research suggests that it may decrease the rate of tooth decay. Chewing sugarless gum increases saliva and thus increases the production of salivary enzymes that help equalize the pH in the mouth and thus reduce cavity growth.

Prevent tooth decay from <u>"morning sickness" by</u>:

a. **Rinsing with a teaspoon of baking soda in a cup of water will neutralize the stomach acids remaining in the mouth after regurgitation.**

b. **Chewing sugarless gum containing xylitol after eating will reduce bacteria and clean teeth without leaving behind cavity-causing sugar.**

Traditionally, mothers-to-be have been reluctant to attend to their dental and oral health needs for fear that diagnostic x-rays and dental procedures could harm their fetus.

The fact is that **untreated oral health problems such as periodontal disease and dental decay are now identified as risk factors for diabetes, dangerously high blood pressure, low birth weight and pre-term delivery**.

Women need to be reassured that it is **now safe** to receive dental care, including digital x-rays and local anesthetics, during all phases of pregnancy. Today's dentists are equipped to provide dental care as an essential component of prenatal care.

NEWBORNS AND DENTAL CARE

After your baby is born, please remember that bacteria can be passed from mother to child. Further, young children should see the dentist at 12 months or after the first tooth erupts into the mouth.

It has been documented that some parents neglect baby teeth because "they are going to fall out anyways." Baby teeth may be small, but they're important. They act as placeholders for adult teeth. Without a healthy set of baby teeth, your child will have trouble chewing and speaking clearly. That's why caring for baby teeth and keeping them decay-free is so important.

You can start caring for your baby's gums right away. But at first, the care won't involve a toothbrush and toothpaste. Instead, take these steps:

- Get a soft, moistened washcloth or piece of gauze.
- Gently wipe down your baby's gums at least twice a day.
- Especially wipe your baby's gums after feedings and before bedtime.

This will wash off bacteria and prevent them from clinging to your baby's gums. Bacteria can leave behind a sticky plaque that damages infant teeth as they erupt.

(a). Brushing Baby's Teeth

When the first baby teeth start to pop up, you can graduate to a toothbrush. Choose one with a:

- Soft brush
- Small head
- Large handle

At first, just wet the toothbrush. At around age 1, you can start using a pea-sized amount of a non-fluoridated toothpaste. **Wait**

to introduce fluoride toothpaste until your child is at least 2 years old. Brush gently all around your child's baby teeth -- front and back.

You should brush your baby's teeth until he or she is old enough to hold the brush. Continue to supervise the process until your child can rinse and spit without assistance. **That usually happens at around age 6.**

Keep on the lookout for any signs of baby tooth decay -- brown or white spots or pits on the teeth. If you or your pediatrician notices any problems, take your child to a dentist for an exam.

(b). Teething

It can take two years before all of the infant teeth have made their way through your baby's gums. The process as each tooth emerges is called "teething." It can be a trying time for you and your baby.

Teething is uncomfortable. That's why your baby cries and fusses in the days or weeks before each baby tooth pops up. Babies can display other teething symptoms, too, including:

- Drooling
- Swollen gums
- Slightly higher than normal temperature

Here are a few tips to relieve your baby's teething pain:

- **Teething rings.** Let your baby chew on a clean, cool teething ring or cold washcloth. Just avoid giving your child anything that is small enough to choke on. Also avoid a teething ring with liquid inside that could break open.
- **Gum rubbing.** Rub your baby's gums with a clean finger.
- **Pain relief.** Give your baby Tylenol (acetaminophen) occasionally to relieve pain -- but ask your pediatrician first. Never give your child aspirin. It has been linked with a rare but serious condition called Reye's syndrome in children.

If your baby is unusually irritable or inconsolable, call your pediatrician.

(c). Preventing Cavities

In addition to caring for baby teeth, you need to protect them. To prevent cavities, only fill your baby's bottle with:

- Formula
- Breast milk
- Water

Avoid giving your child fruit juices, sodas, and other sugary drinks. Sweet drinks -- even milk -- can settle on the teeth. This can lead to baby tooth decay -- also known as "baby bottle tooth decay." Bacteria feed on the sugar from sweet drinks and produce acid, which attacks your baby's teeth.

If you have to send your baby to bed or naps with a bottle or Sippy cup, fill it with water only. Also avoid putting anything sweet — such as sugar or honey — on your baby's pacifier.

SUMMARY

Being Pregnant is a very exciting time in your life. Be sure to consider your overall and dental health and provide an optimum environment for your unborn child and soon to be newborn!

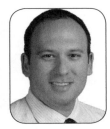

About Dr. Frank Orlando

Frank Orlando, DDS, FAGD, FICOI maintains a private dental office in Midtown Manhattan focused on Comprehensive Cosmetic and Implant Dentistry with a specific focus on Oral Systemic Health. He strives to educate patients on oral health - as an integral part to systemic health. He is focused on patient comfort and care and provides a relaxed setting with the most advanced technology to provide his patients with optimum conservative and long-term treatment.

As a founding member of the **American Academy of Oral Systemic Health** and a **Fellow in the Academy of General Dentistry** and **The International Congress of Oral Implantologists,** Dr. Orlando is well-versed in all aspects of general and advanced dentistry with a continual focus on improving your oral health to optimize your overall systemic health.

For a free list of oral and dental health DO's and DON'Ts for new mothers and mothers-to-be, or to receive a complimentary oral health consultation, women who are pregnant or in the planning stages may contact:
Frank Orlando, DDS, FAGD, FICOI
24 West 57th Street, Suite 701
New York, NY 10019
(646) 926-7402
drfrankorlando@gmail.com
www.drfrankorlando.com

CHAPTER 10

HEALTHY GUMS, HEALTHY BODY: THE POWER OF LASER TREATMENTS

MICHAEL FRITH, DDS, FAGD

Now, more than ever, we understand that what happens in one part of our body can have a profound effect on the rest of our health. Also, we understand how our bodies are a very connected system - and *all* parts need to be functioning at their best for us to function at our best.

Nowhere is that more true than with, believe it or not, our gums.

It's only been in the last ten or twenty years, that science has discovered just how critical good oral health is to your complete well-being. Gum disease (or periodontal disease) can actually be a trigger for some other very serious illnesses in the rest of your body (including your mouth). After all, gum disease is the number one cause of tooth loss, beating tooth decay by a two-to-one margin.

In this chapter, I'm going to discuss in depth just how untreated gum disease can pose a significant danger to your overall health – and how a new hi-tech treatment can easily prevent that danger and keep your gums in great shape without any pain or discomfort.

I. THE FACTS ABOUT GUM DISEASE

Gum disease is taken so seriously these days that some physicians, before they'll do certain surgeries such as heart transplants and hip replacements, will require that the patient have their dentist sign off on their oral health before they'll perform the operation.

To quote a *Wall Street Journal* article from December 27th, 2011, *"There's growing evidence that oral health problems, particularly gum disease, can harm a patient's general health as well, raising the risk of diabetes, heart disease, stroke, pneumonia and pregnancy complications."* In that same article, Anthony Iacopino, Director of the International Centre for Oral-Systemic Health, says, *"We have lots of data showing a direct correlation between inflammation in the mouth and inflammation in the body."*

What causes gum disease? Plaque buildup on teeth happens to all of us and is why gum disease is so common; around 75% of American adults suffer from gum disease at some point in their lives, with almost 30% showing the symptoms of more severe gum disease, chronic periodontitis.

You might be asking, "How can my gums possibly affect the rest of my body?" Well, gum disease causes a lot of bad bacteria to be present in your mouth. Also, your gums become swollen and more blood gets into them – which is why they bleed when you suffer from gum disease and you brush your teeth. When your gums bleed, guess what? The door is open for the bacteria on your gums to enter your blood stream, where it can attach to blood vessels and increase clot formations. Other organs are then at risk.

Let's look more closely at a few of the health concerns that gum disease can trigger.

- **Heart Disease**
  Believe it or not, research done by The American Heart Association shows that poor oral health increases the likelihood of heart disease by an even greater degree

than high cholesterol and triglyceride levels do.

As already noted, gum disease can lead to blood clots, which can end up decreasing the blood supply flow to the heart and increasing the chances of a heart attack. One study done in America analyzed the data for almost ten thousand people. That study found that those with periodontitis had a 25% increased risk of coronary heart disease compared to those with little or no periodontal disease. For males under the age of fifty, periodontal disease was an even bigger risk factor – they had nearly *twice* the risk of coronary heart disease than men who had little or no gum disease.

- **Diabetes**
  Gum disease can actually induce diabetes as well. That same bacteria from your mouth doesn't just cause clots, it can also activate your immune cells. Once activated, these cells then produce inflammatory biological signals called "cytokines" that can have a very harsh effect throughout your entire body.

And when it comes to diabetes, the cells in your pancreas that are responsible for insulin production can be damaged or even destroyed by chronic high levels of cytokines. And that's where Type 2 diabetes can happen — even in otherwise healthy individuals with no other risk factors for diabetes. If you are already diabetic, good oral care becomes critical. The problems controlling blood sugar caused by both Type 1 and Type 2 diabetes affect the mouth in various ways, including:

(a) Dry Mouth: Increased blood sugar can lead to a decrease in saliva, causing dry mouth.

(b) Gum Disease: Yes, even if gum disease helped create the diabetes, the diabetes can come right back and worsen the gum disease. Diabetes cuts down on our ability to fight infections, so it's easier for the bacteria normally present in the mouth to over-whelm those defenses and for gum disease to become more severe.

(c) Slow Healing: Diabetes reduces blood flow, so it's more difficult for the mouth to heal after oral surgery.

(d) Thrush: The high levels of sugar found in diabetic saliva – along with decreased resistance – can lead to this fungal infection in the mouth.

For these reasons and more, it's especially important for diabetics to see their dentists regularly. A dentist will often work with a diabetic patient's medical doctor to come up with a care plan that works for them. This means knowing what medications the patient is currently taking, being aware of the patient's blood sugar levels during treatments, and taking their condition into account when scheduling any oral surgery or other serious procedures.

- **Cancer**
  The link between cancer and gum disease is undeniable; a British and American research team at Imperial College in London and Harvard University studied the statistical health records of fifty thousand patients from data collected over twenty-one years. Those that suffered from gum disease had a 33% increase in the risk of lung cancer, a 50% rise in the risk of kidney cancer, and a 30% higher incidence of blood cancers, such as leukemia.

When the gum disease was chronic, the link grew even stronger and more frightening: there was an additional *fourfold* increase in head and neck cancer for each millimeter of related bone loss around the teeth.

Another recent study by the Dana-Farber Cancer Institute and the Harvard School of Public Health established a strong link between periodontal disease and pancreatic cancer. The study, eliminating all risk factors for pancreatic cancer (such as age, body mass index, smoking, etc.), discovered that those with gum disease were *63% more likely* to develop pancreatic cancer than those who didn't have periodontal disease.

What's the scientific explanation of this? Again, it comes down to bacteria from the mouth getting into the bloodstream and causing inflammation. This inflammation could theoretically promote the growth of cancer cells, but this is an area that is still being researched.

- **<u>Chronic Bad Breath</u>**
  I think you'll agree that bad breath isn't anywhere near as serious as heart disease or cancer – but you'll also probably agree that bad breath can make your life miserable in a myriad of other ways, as hundreds of TV commercials over the years have demonstrated. Whether at work, at a social engagement or even just home with friends and family, bad breath, medically known as halitosis, can lead to constant embarrassment and avoidance of any close contact with others.

Bad breath is caused by bacteria, which break down proteins already in the mouth. These proteins, and other materials which are in the mouth either naturally or from what we eat and drink, are the real power behind bad breath. As, I've already noted, gum disease creates an abundance of bacteria that easily creates the conditions for halitosis to happen.

If you continue to have bad breath after you've brushed and flossed (and scraped your tongue), gum disease is the most likely culprit. And considering everything you've learned so far about what gum disease can do to the rest of your body, you should definitely visit your dentist to take care of it.

II. TREATING GUM DISEASE

Obviously, to prevent gum disease, you should practice as much good oral hygiene as possible – that, of course, includes regular brushing and flossing. You may still, however, be susceptible to gum disease even if you do take good care of your teeth – research shows that almost a third of the population is genetically predisposed to gum disease and may be up to six times more likely to develop periodontal disease. That's why visiting a dentist on a regular basis is important, because you never know when gum disease may occur and you want to treat it at as early a stage as possible. Again, tooth loss is yet another common problem that could develop as a result of failing to deal with the problem.

In the past, there were basically only two options when it came to treating gum disease, besides preventative maintenance:

(1) Performing a deep cleaning on the teeth to clean out plaque and pockets of bacteria, and, in more severe cases,

(2) Periodontal surgery, in which a gum specialist (a periodontist) will actually cut away part of the gum and clean out the infected area. More recently, antibiotics have also been utilized to treat these kinds of infections.

In recent years, however, I (and other dentists as well) have offered patients what I consider to be an amazing new alternative – *laser periodontal treatment*.

Gum surgery can be painful, slow to heal and can also leave you with the lower parts of your teeth exposed, because of the removal of parts of your gum. Even a deep cleaning can be an extremely uncomfortable and lengthy process, depending on how much periodontal disease is present.

Initially, a normal cleaning is needed where the plaque (with its biofilm) and hard tartar are removed. Then this is where the laser treatment brings many advantages. It's the only treatment that can disinfect and decontaminate deeper gum pockets. Merely scraping the roots of the teeth can't do either of these. It can be done quickly, painlessly and relatively inexpensively. It's not invasive, as surgery and even a deep cleaning can be, and yet, a laser can still reach hidden areas that a normal cleaning can't access. Research has also shown that laser decontamination is more effective than antibiotics at killing bacteria. Some bacteria are resistant to drugs – no bacteria can withstand the laser treatment. Antibiotics also can suppress your immune system and create resistance to medicines you might need at a later time for a more serious need.

Any possible discomfort you might experience with a laser treatment is eliminated by the use of a topical anesthetic. Laser treatment also has a much quicker recovery time than periodontal surgery and also costs less. There are other benefits associated with laser treatments as well, such as improving your breath, and reducing the risk of diabetes, due to the gum bacteria factors I discussed earlier. If you are already diabetic, it can greatly increase your life expectancy by, again, eliminating bacteria and the risk of infections.

III. CASE STUDIES

From my professional standpoint, having been in dentistry for over thirty years, I've been amazed at the positive effect laser treatment has had in controlling and preventing gum disease. Lasers in your mouth may sound like science fiction, but it's actually a very gentle procedure that helps you avoid much more intensive procedures, such as surgery. Laser treatments may also mean you may not even need the services of a periodontist.

I'd like to end this chapter by talking about what laser treatment has done for a couple of my patients. Vicki, a sixty year-old woman who works in sales, has been coming in for treatment at my dental practice for over twenty-five years. According to her, "All my experience before was hating to go to the dentist because it was miserable and it hurt so bad. Since I went to you, it hasn't been that way."

Vicki had a lot of gum problems that were causing her problems. "I thought I could just keep going to the dentist and it would go away – but I realized I needed to do something extra to take care of it." Since she began laser treatments, she no longer needed to consult with a specialist. "Your office does everything the gum specialist did for me. I have not been to that office since you started using the laser on me. I'm sure it's helping in the deepest areas where stuff gets caught. The laser treatment is also easy and not painful at all."

Then there's John, who is 48 years old and works in an IT capacity at a healthcare company. John's been coming to our office for about fifteen years, ever since his wisdom teeth were causing him problems.

"I had impacted wisdom teeth, so you referred me to an oral surgeon for their removal. After that, I returned to your office and you told me I had gum disease. I did begin to notice some loose teeth and that my gums were receding. I started getting laser treatment from you a few years ago. The topical numbing did the trick and the treatment wasn't uncomfortable at all, I only felt a warming sensation that wasn't painful. Gum bleeding would slow after every treatment and improvement was evident – it was a lot better than losing more teeth. It was definitely one of the turning points in getting things under control. My gums are definitely healthier."

Those are just two of the many happy results laser treatment has provided to my patients. There are many others who would report similar positive outcomes.

Gum disease is a serious matter. Treating it, however, doesn't have to be a big ordeal. Laser treatment is quick, convenient, painless and provides long-lasting benefits. If you're suffering from gum problems, I suggest you talk to a dental professional who can provide this service to see if it might be right for you.

About Dr. Michael Frith

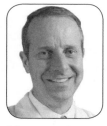

Michael Frith, DDS, FAGD is one of the most trusted and progressive dentists in St. Louis. For over 30 years, he has passionately dedicated his life to his profession, his family and his faith. While growing up in Iowa, he decided to pursue the health professions. After earning a BS degree from the University of Iowa, he also attended dental school there, where he received his DDS degree in 1979. Seeking the best opportunity for growth, he (and his wife, Julie) moved to St. Louis in 1981 to build a dynamic private practice.

Dr. Frith contributed his time for many years to dental leadership, and in 1995 served as the President of the West County District of the Greater St. Louis Dental Society. Since then, he has been extremely involved in dental education and received his Accreditation award from the American Academy of Cosmetic Dentistry and Fellowship award from the Academy of General Dentistry.

He currently holds membership in important dental organizations such as the American Dental Association, Missouri Dental Association, Greater St. Louis Dental Society, International Association of Orthodontics, Academy of General Dentistry, American Academy of Cosmetic Dentistry, American Academy of Dental Sleep Medicine, and the American Academy of Craniofacial Pain. He is also the Director of the TMJ and Sleep Therapy Centre of St. Louis.

Dr. Frith owns and uses six different lasers on a daily basis. In recent years, Dr. Frith and his wife have been 'giving back' by serving in different third world countries on dental mission trips.